The Practice Nurse

The Practice Nurse
Theory and practice

Pauline Jeffree

SPRINGER-SCIENCE+BUSINESS MEDIA, B.V.

First edition 1990

© 1990 Pauline Jeffree

Originally published by Chapman and Hall in 1990

Typeset in 10 on 12 pt Sabon by
Best-set Typesetter Ltd, Hong Kong

ISBN 978-0-412-33590-7

British Library Cataloguing in Publication Data

Jeffree, Pauline
  1. The practice nurse: theory and practice.
  1. General practice. Nursing
  I. Title
  610.73

ISBN 978-0-412-33590-7   ISBN 978-1-4899-6876-0 (eBook)
DOI 10.1007/978-1-4899-6876-0

Library of Congress Cataloging in Publication Data

available

To my Colleagues
at Elm House Surgery

Contents

Acknowledgements

This book for Practice Nurses would not have been written without the inspiration and encouragement of Dr Peter Jarvis.

I would especially like to mention the following, to whom I am indebted: Dr Kenneth Scott, who not only contributed to the text, but also personally offered constant encouragement and support and whose comments have considerably enriched the text. Dr John Fry, who patiently and painstakingly shared with me the writing of the book and who kindly agreed to contribute a chapter to the book. Practice Nurse students who have helped me to clarify issues in our learning and teaching sessions at the University of Surrey and North East Surrey College of Technology.

I would like to express my gratitude to those who have kindly given permission to reproduce from other sources. In the final analysis, however, the ultimate responsibility for the content of the book must rest with the author.

Preface

It is anticipated over the next few years that there will be major developments in the provision of service in community and primary care. This changing philosophy of care will place great demands on the Primary Care Team.

The Practice Nurse in particular will have a major role to play in the changing and expanding spectrum of primary health care provision.

This book seeks to provide the theory and its practical application for Practice Nurse colleagues as we face the exciting challenges of the future and move forward with the Government's White Paper *Working for Patients*.

Pauline Jeffree

Foreword

A new concept of care has emerged in recent years with the introduction of nurses into General Practice working alongside General Practitioners in surgeries and health centres.

Significant changes have occurred in both primary and community care with the changing philosophy of health provision and the introduction of 'Care in the Community'. This has further been compounded by a reduction of hospital services in some Districts and a shorter length of stay which has made greater demands for the Primary Care Team in General Practice.

The attachment of Community Nurses to General Practices has not met the entire needs of the developing services and an increasing number of General Practitioners are employing their own Practice Nurse. The skills required by the Nurse in General Practice are numerous and varied, not only to meet the needs of the practice population but also to make an essential contribution to the Primary Care Team.

The author of this book has had the foresight to realize that at the present time there are nurses who need guidance and information about the tasks they are expected to carry out in the surgery or health centre and she has covered a very wide spectrum of care programmes and procedures in a very comprehensive way.

She has also given well deserved space in the book to advise nurses about the ethics and legalities with which a nurse in practice can be involved.

At the time of going to press the Government's White Paper *Working for Patients* clearly indicates their expectations of a greater spectrum of health care, including treatment, surveillance and health promotion in General Practice. This can only be achieved by strengthening Primary Care Teams and developing their professional skills in General Practice.

Practice Nurses have a major contribution to make to the development of primary care and the purpose of this book is to equip them with the basic knowledge to provide that care.

Kenneth Scott MB, BS, FRCGP, DRCOG
General Practitioner, Beckenham, Kent.
General Manager,
Community and Mental Handicap Unit,
Bromley Health Authority,
Kent.

1

The National Health Service – history and reorganization

Dr Kenneth Scott MB, BS, FRCGP, DRCOG
Senior Partner,
Elm House Surgery, Kent

HEALTH CARE BEFORE THE ESTABLISHMENT OF THE NHS

There is probably no single strand in the history of health care in the United Kingdom that can be identified as the origin of the National Health Service (NHS). Our first recognized hospital was founded by monks in Smithfield, London in the 12th century.

Subsequent improvements in social conditions are linked to the development of health care, the origins of which were formulated in the 16th century with the introduction of the first Poor Law Act (1569) during the reign of Elizabeth I. It was recognized at that time that provision had to be made for the vagrants, the destitute, the elderly and the insane.

The establishment of county asylums for the insane and ward provision for the destitute sick came some three centuries later with the passing of the County Asylums Act (1809).

Significant improvements in the welfare of the poor evolved slowly, both through various amendments to the Poor Law and Government Reform Acts (1834, 1867) and through improved sanitation, standards of living and diet.

Some infectious diseases seemed to lose their virulence and deaths from such conditions as smallpox, plague and typhus gradually diminished.

Medical knowledge, which had stagnated for centuries, made

great strides forward with the development of diagnostic skills, the meticulous observation of the physicians of the day, improved surgical techniques and such major events as the development of the microscope, the discovery of anaesthetics and the use of medication. Improved medical education followed, which brought in its wake greater improvements in medical skills.

By the late 18th century and during the 19th century clinical conditions could be treated more effectively which resulted in a complete revolution in the use and function of hospitals. They changed their role from establishments to care for the elderly infirm and insane to centres where treatments and surgical procedures could be carried out. At this time hospitals were still established and maintained by religious or charitable organizations, voluntary bodies, local councils and by the generosity of individuals. During the 19th century physicians and surgeons took more meaningful posts in established hospitals, mostly in an honorary capacity, and no longer treated their patients at home which until this time was the custom. In 1848 the General Board of Health was established.

General Practice, unique to the United Kingdom, must have its origins from the physicians, surgeons and apothecaries who remained exclusively in the community to consult and treat the local population.

THE NATIONAL HEALTH SERVICE

Three major events led to the establishment of the NHS. The first of these events was the Royal Commission at the beginning of this century which lead to the National Insurance Act (1911) identifying the basic structure of General Practice for the working population.

The second event was the Local Government Act (1929) which transferred responsibility for health care to local authorities who mainly provided care in the community.

The third event, the Beveridge Report (1942), was designed to review social service provision in the United Kingdom. In the context of the Report the recommendation was made to establish a NHS funded mainly by direct tax providing medical treatment for all citizens without charge. In 1946 the National Health Service Act was passed and the NHS was established on the 5th July, 1948.

The Ministry of Health, founded in 1919, was responsible for the

NHS from 1948–68 when it was absorbed into the Department of Health and Social Security.

However, in 1989, the Departments were again separated and the post of Secretary of State for Health was created.

The first glimmer of co-operation between General Practitioners and District Nurses came with the Dawson Report (1920) which recommended the development of primary and secondary care by the establishment of health centres where doctors and nurses could work together for the benefit of their patients.

At the onset of the NHS a tri-partite structure* was established to satisfy the resistance of many professional groups and professional organizations; with considerable disappointment by some that the hospital services were not to be included in local authority administration. The hospital services were nationalized and administered by some 400 Management Committees who were responsible to 15 Regional Health Boards.

The Teaching Hospitals, however, were given special consideration and were controlled by separate Teaching Hospital Boards.

Resulting from negotiations with the Minister of Health, the General Medical Services Committee became the General Practitioner's representative body.

The General Practitioner, Dental Surgeon, Ophthalmic and Pharmaceutical services were to be administered by newly established Executive Councils. The professionals within these services were to be recognized as independent contractors to the NHS.

In addition to the Hospital Service and the Primary Care under Executive Councils; the third arm of this complex structure was the health care that remained under the administration of local authorities and this included all community nursing provision. District Nurses, Health Visitors and Community Midwives were responsible to the Medical Officer of Health. The local authority also retained responsibility for the school health service, public health provision and the ambulance service.

---

* Tri-partite structure:
   Hospital Groups, responsible to Regional Health Authorities;
   Executive Councils, to whom General Practitioners, District Pharmicists,
   Opticians and Dentists were responsible;
   Local Authorities, responsible for provision of county medical and nursing staff
   such as District Nurses, Health Visitors, School Nurses and Midwives; and who
   were responsible to the Medical Health Officer.

The immediate result was that everyone residing in the UK was entitled to free health care from all branches of the NHS from General Practice, local authority and hospital services.

In the post-war years medical and surgical skills developed and new techniques were introduced. Treatments that had hitherto only been dreamed about were coming to fruition. The Health Service expanded rapidly and costs escalated.

FIRST REORGANIZATION, 1974

To meet the needs of the developing service it was recognized in the early 1960s that the management of the NHS was less than ideal and that reorganization was necessary. The first reorganization took place, after several Government Green Papers, in 1974. Major changes were implemented and perhaps the most significant was that local authorities were eliminated from the health scene; they were no longer responsible for community medical and nursing care but did, however, continue to provide environmental services.

This reorganization had important implications for primary care services. The 138 Executive Councils were replaced by some 90 Family Practitioner Committees who were staffed by Health Authorities but still had direct responsibility to the Secretary of State for Health and Social Services.

Hospital services were restructured and hospital groups were re-structured to create 206 District Health Authorities responsible to Area Health Authorities who in their turn were responsible to 14 Regional Health Authorities and Teaching Hospital Boards. The Area Health Authorities were largely responsible for planning and covered either single or multiple Districts.

Management Teams were established to manage the Areas and Districts and were responsible to their Area and District Health Authorities and, with their introduction, consensus management was introduced into the NHS.

Each Team consisted of six members of an Area or District: a Nursing Officer, Administrator, Medical Officer, Treasurer, one Consultant, and one General Practitioner representing their colleagues.

A further significant development in this reorganization was the establishment of:

1. *Community Health Councils* – these organizations were
   established in each District to represent the general public and
   ensure that local views were conveyed to the Health Authorities.
   They have the right to challenge major changes in the provision
   of service and are in a position to offer alternative plans which
   have to be considered by the Health Authority; where there is
   disagreement the Authorities have the right of appeal to the
   Secretary of State;
2. *Joint Consultative Committees* – these were created to
   encourage the integration of local authority and Social Services'
   provision with the Health Authority and to develop care
   programmes in the community.

Shortly after the first reorganization came the introduction of the
recommendations of the Resource Allocation Working Party
(RAWP) (1978/1979) whose aim was to equate health care provision across the country. Funds were transferred from the more
affluent regions to regions whose services needed to be expanded
and transferred from district to district from within the same
region. Shares of NHS resources were based on population, mortality, morbidity and hospital bed utilization – rates in accordance
with the RAWP formula which aimed at providing similar services
to all districts. However, in exercising this new approach the
London and Oxford Regions have been reduced in their funding
which has had a significant effect on the development of the
Teaching Hospitals in London. This may in turn have damaging
long-term effects on these centres of excellence.

Within a few years of reorganization it was recognized that
further changes were needed to develop the NHS. Each District
wanted further autonomy in managing its affairs and wanted direct
access to its parent Regional Health Authority.

SECOND REORGANIZATION, 1982

In 1982 the second reorganization took place, the essential feature
of which was elimination of the Area Health Authority. The 90
AHAs and 206 DHAs were reduced to 192 DHAs each responsible
to its own RHA or Special Health Authority.

As part of this rearrangement, it was planned that FPCs should
be independent of HAs. This occurred in 1985. They now receive

direct funding from the DHSS thus ensuring FPC independence, but are subject to the DHSS review process and perhaps greater directing of services.

The reorganizations of 1974 and 1982 aimed to review the cumbersome structure and reduce the number of Districts. Each District being more autonomous yet the Regional Health Authority holding the purse strings. These developments gave greater possibility for the public to be aware of and to criticize their health service through the CHC. DHA's became responsible for medical and nursing and community services so that care in the community could be a reality.

The implementation of RAWP, designed to equate health provision across the country, was being felt in the well provided areas. To achieve District financial targets a massive bed reduction was under way both for acute and long stay beds which has caused a greater need for community provision.

The ability to reduce hospital beds is linked with the development of medical nursing and other professional skills in the diagnosis and treatment of many acute clinical conditions. Development of intensive care and coronary care units plays an important role in improving treatment and consequently shortening the length of stay in hospital.

Development and care of the elderly must not be overlooked, and the need for better housing, diet, activity and general stimulation and increased mobility may well have reduced the incidence of chronic disabling illness in the elderly.

During the late 1970s and early 1980s new thinking was emerging about the care of people with mental handicap and mental illness. It was no longer considered appropriate that people with such conditions should be incarcerated in institutions. Developments in programmes of care and medication would enable these patients to be cared for in the community and thus the Priority Care Groups became established with the aim of closing all long stay institutions.

It was apparent in 1982/1983 that although the NHS reorganization had restructured the service, it had done little to improve the management arrangements. Management was laborious and decisions took too long to make and much longer to implement. In response to this situation, the Prime Minister commissioned Roy Griffiths to look at the management of the NHS and recommend a new, more effective structure.

THE GRIFFITHS REPORT

1983 saw the publication of the Griffiths Report and its almost, in NHS terms, immediate implementation. Region and District Health Authority structure remained. District Management Teams were eliminated and with them consensus management. District Management Boards were created and were responsible to DHAs. Each District was autonomous in setting up its own Unit structure to provide its services.

Each Unit had its own Manager responsible to the District General Manager who in turn was responsible to the Regional General Manager.

The management of the NHS was taken over by the NHS Board responsible to the Secretary of State who is accountable to Parliament.

The Griffiths concept of management in the NHS had very important implications for the Community Services. All Districts have a Community or Priority Care Unit with its own Manager. The opportunity is there to integrate community and Primary Care under its own Unit of Management, with its own administration, finance and resource staff with control of its own budget and the facility to exercise virement within the Unit.

The Unit Management structure envisaged by Griffiths was to devolve Management responsibility to the lowest level within the Unit that was capable of accepting it and with this management responsibility it is intended to transfer the Budgetary control.

The Community Unit is ideal to demonstrate this new concept of responsibilities in that each Community Unit could be securized, each Sector having its own Manager who would be in a position to determine the local needs in the Sector and holding the budget they will have the facility to rearrange services to meet the specific needs of that particular Sector in the District.

The door is open for Community Managers to work closely with the (independent) FPCs to integrate the social, community and Primary Care Services, in which the Practice Nurse has an ever expanding role.

At the time of this publication we anxiously await the Government's view on the recently published Griffiths Report on Community Services (1988).

The White Paper *Working for Patients* (January, 1989) has given recommendations for the future organization and management of the Community Health Services.

This White Paper entitled *Working for Patients* has proposed a new concept of care within the Health Service and has major implications for both primary and secondary care. The Government has invited Hospitals within the NHS to become self-governing and for General Practitioners working in large Practices of not less than 11 000 patients to hold their own budgets to purchase some services for their patients from hospitals that can offer them the best contract. A further development contained in this document has removed the independence of the Family Practitioner Committees who are, after 1990, under the responsibility of Regional Health Authorities. The Government's proposals are intended to take effect between 1990 and 1993.

The basic principles of the Government's White Paper identifies that patients' needs are paramount and they should have the extended choice of all services and that these services should remain free at the point of delivery. District Health Authorities should be responsible for meeting the health needs of their local population.

There are many unsolved issues, not least the continuing care of priority care groups and the question of whose ultimate responsibility it will be to develop integration of Primary, Community and Social Services to meet the needs of the Community.

In conclusion, it can be said that the NHS has made great strides since its inception. Forty years have seen outstanding developments in medical and nursing skills, investigation techniques and treatments. Improved social conditions and health provision are enabling people to live longer, and both physically and mentally handicapped as well as the mentally ill will be taking their rightful place in our communities.

FURTHER READING

Abel-Smith, B. (1964) *The Hospitals 1800–1948*, Heinemann Educational Books, London.

Klein, R. (1983) *The Politics of the National Health Service*, Longman, Harlow.

Pater, J.E. (1981) *The Making of the National Health Service*, Kings Fund, London.

Titmus, R.M. (1950) *Problems of Social Policy*, London.

Taylor, D. (1984) *Understanding the NHS in the 1980s*, Office of Health Economics, 12, Whitehall, London, SW1A 2DY.

Appendix

Reports

DHSS (1976a) *Priorities for Health and Social Services in England*, HMSO, London.
DHSS (1976b) *Sharing Resources for Health in England*, HMSO, London.
DHSS (1976d) *Prevention and Health: Everybody's Business*, HMSO, London.
DHSS (1977) *The Way Forward*, HMSO, London.
DHSS (1979) *Patients First*, HMSO, London.
DHSS (1980) *Inequalities in Health (Black Reports)*, DHSS, London.
DHSS (1981a) *Care in Action*, HMSO, London.
DHSS (1981b) *Care in the Community*, DHSS, London.
DHSS (1983) *Health Care and its Costs*, HMSO, London.
Social Services Committee (1984) *Griffiths, R. Report: NHS Management*, HMSO, London.

2

Primary health care – what is it and who does it?

Dr John Fry CBE, MD, FRCS, FRCGP
Principal in General Practice and Senior Partner, Beckenham, Kent

HEALTH CARE

Health care is a basic human right. It has to be provided in some form or other in all societies.

The form and range of health care depend on many factors such as national health, politics, religion, customs, geography, climate and resources.

The demands for care are infinite. The resources are finite. So everywhere there have to be limits, restrictions, priorities and rationing. The challenges are to make the most use of available resources.

SYSTEMS

There are four national systems of health care world-wide:

- a private free enterprise system as in the USA, West Germany and Japan;
- a socialized system as in the USSR, Eastern Europe, Cuba and China;
- a mix of public and private systems as in the UK, Scandinavia, Netherlands, Australia, and New Zealand;
- a 'no system' system in countries too poor to create a comprehensive national system.

Levels of health care

Within all systems of health care there are four recognizable levels of care relating to who does it and where, the population size and administration.

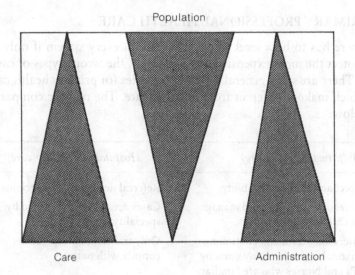

Self care

This level relates to health care carried out by the individual and family members or within a family unit of 1–10 persons.

Primary professional care

This refers to health care at the level of General Practice (in the UK) but the person of first contact may be a Doctor, Nurse, Social Worker or Hospital Unit. The base is a neighbourhood of 2000–10 000 persons depending on area and service.

General specialties secondary care

This category relates to health care carried out by General Surgeons, Physicians, OBG's, Paediatricians, Psychiatrists, etc., all based at a District General Hospital caring for around 250 000 persons.

Super specialist tertiary care

Lastly, this type of care is available from Regional Units such as Cardiothoracic, Neurological, Renal Dialysis, etc., covering a population of 1–5 million.

PRIMARY PROFESSIONAL HEALTH CARE

There has to be a level of primary care in every system if only to protect the more expensive hospitals from the wrong types of case.

There are some general features and roles for primary health care which make it different from hospital care. The two are compared below:

GP (primary health care)	Hospital (secondary care)
Direct access and availability	Referral needed to see specialist
GP team must assess and manage the case from the start	Cases are already presented by speciality
Offers long-term and continuing personal care over many years by GPs and Nurses who are familiar with the patient	Only transient and episodic contact with patients
Population cared for is relatively small – about 2000 per GP	A District General Hospital covers a population of some 250 000
Common conditions occur commonly and rare conditions rarely	Rare conditions are more common

THE GENERAL PRACTICE MODEL

There are over 30 000 General Practitioners in the NHS who work from about 10 000 practice units.

The following model shows a typical GP team for a practice population of 10 000:

- 3–4 GP Principals;
- 1 or 2 GP Trainees;
- 1 Practice Manager/Administrator;
- 5–6 Full-time Receptionists or 10–15 part-time Receptionists;

- 1 Practice Nurse;
- 2–3 attached District Nurses;
- 1–2 attached Health Visitors;
- 1 attached Midwife;
- possibly others such as Social Workers, Psychologists, Counsellors, etc.

ORGANIZATION OF GENERAL PRACTICE

There is a continuing trend towards larger practices so that the single-handed GP is now a rarity, whereas when the NHS started in 1948 about one half of all GPs worked in single practices.

The distribution of GPs by practice size is now:

Number of GPs in practice	% of GPs
1	11
2	16
3	21
4	19
5	15
6 and over	18

WORK PATTERNS

The GP's work largely consists of consultations in the surgery or in practice clinics, and home visits.

The facts on work in General Practice are as follows:

- average list size per GP is 2000 patients;
- about two-thirds of all persons will consult their GP once or more per year;
- the average annual patient consultation rate (surgery and home visits) is 3–4. This means that a GP with 2000 patients can expect 6000–8000 consultations in a year;
- an average surgery consultation is 5–10 minutes;
- an average home visit takes 20–30 minutes, including travel time.

A typical week in hours spent can be illustrated as follows:

Type of work	Hours per week
Surgery consultations	16
Home visits	14
Clinics	1
Paperwork and discussions over patients	5
Administration	2
Teaching	1
Other	1
Total hours	40

In addition he/she may be 'on call' for 30 hours.

CONTENT OF WORK

The type of work of General Practice mirrors the complaints that will occur in a population of say 10 000 which is the size of an average group of 4–5 GPs which will employ a Practice Nurse.

Happenings per year	Per population of 10 000
Births	130
Deaths	
Cardiac	41
Cancer	21
Respiratory	21
Strokes	15
Accidents, etc.	8
Others	9
Total deaths	115

Most of the clinical work in General Practice is with minor and chronic disorders:

Minor	60%
Chronic	30%
Major (acute)	10%

In order of frequency the most prevalent **minor conditions** are:

- respiratory and ENT;
- skin;
- rheumatic;
- psycho-emotional;
- gastro-intestinal;
- gynaecological and urinary;
- accidents.

The likely annual prevalence of **chronic conditions** per GP with 2000 patients is given below by numbers of patients consulting:

High blood pressure	80
Asthma and chronic bronchitis	55
Osteoarthritis	50
Chronic depression, etc.	45
Heart failure	45
Peptic ulcers	12
Strokes (aftercare)	12
Rheumatoid disease	10
Epilepsy	7
Parkinsonism	3
Multiple sclerosis	2

The annual prevalence of **acute major disease** per GP with 2000 patients will be:

Acute bronchitis/pneumonia	20
Acute myocardial infarction	10
New cancers	7
Acute strokes	5

A considerable amount of work in general practice is now concerned with **non-illness** and the numbers of persons seen per year in a practice of 2000 will be:

Family planning	115
Immunizations	100
Medical check-ups, insurance, certification, etc.	50
Cervical cytology	50
Antenatal/postnatal	40

Of importance but not necessarily involving the practice is the social pathology that exists in the population. In an average population of 2000 there are:

- 175 persons on supplementary allowances;
- 100 unemployed;
- 50 handicapped;
- 12 marriages per year;
- 5 divorces per year;
- 5 illegitimate births per year;
- 4 terminations of pregnancy per year;
- 400 smokers;
- 300 heavy drinkers;
- 36 burglaries per year;
- 5 personal assaults per year;
- 1 sexual offence per year;
- 2 persons in prison;
- 4 children in care;
- 10 juvenile delinquents.

COST OF GENERAL PRACTICE

The NHS is not free. The annual cost in 1987 was £390 per person per year or approximately £22 billion.

About one quarter of the NHS budget is spent annually (1987) on general practice.

Each GP is responsible for over £200 000 of NHS expenditure per year.

FURTHER READING

Geyman, J.P. and Fry, J. (1983) *Family Practice: an International Perspective in Developed Countries*, Appleton-Century-Croft, Norwalk, Conn., USA.

Dopson, L. (1971) *The Changing Scene in General Practice*, Johnson, London.

Gibson, R. (1981) *The Family Doctor: His Life and History*, George Allen and Unwin, London.

Fry, J. (1988) *GP Data Book*, MTP, Lancaster.

Fry, J. (1985) *Common Diseases* (4th Edn), MTP, Lancaster.

Stephen, W.J. (1979) *An Analysis of Primary Medical Care*, Cambridge University Press, Cambridge.

Jefferys, M. and Sachs, H. (1983) *Rethinking General Practice*, Tavistock, London.

Reedy, B.L.E.C. (1980) in *Primary Care* (Ed. J. Fry), Heinemann, London.

DHSS (1987) *Health and Personal Social Services Statistics*, HMSO, London.

Fry, J. (1988) *General Practice and Primary Health Care, 1940–1980*. The Nuffield Provincial Hospitals Trust.

3

Ethics and training

NURSING ETHICS

In law, each person is responsible for his/her own actions and the reasonable consequences of those actions.

In ethics, the action of a competent member of the medical profession is measured by similar medical practitioners. These practitioners sit in judgement.

Guidance for Nurses, Midwives and Health Visitors is laid down in the UKCC's Code of Professional Conduct. These Rules provide guidance on normal, acceptable professional behaviour.

In nursing, the National Boards for England, Scotland, Wales and Northern Ireland assess whether an infringement of the Rules has occurred. If an infringement is indeed thought to have occurred the United Kingdom Central Council (UKCC) will give full consideration of the complaint through the Professional Conduct Committee.

CODE OF PROFESSIONAL CONDUCT

The Code of Professional Conduct for Nurses, Midwives and Health Visitors (based on ethical concepts) has no legal standing but states:

> 'Each registered Nurse, Midwife and Health Visitor shall act, at all times, in such a manner as to justify public trust and confidence, to uphold and enhance the good standing and reputation of the profession, to serve the interests of the society, and above all to safeguard the interests of individual patients and clients.'

The Code further states that 'Each Registered Nurse, Midwife and Health Visitor is accountable for his or her practice, and, in the exercise of professional accountability shall:

1. Always act in such a way as to promote and safeguard the well being and interests of patients/clients;
2. Ensure that no action or omission on his/her part or within his/her sphere of influence is detrimental to the condition or safety of patients/clients;
3. Take every reasonable opportunity to maintain and improve professional knowledge and competence;
4. Acknowledge any limitations of competence and refuse in such cases to accept delegated functions without first having received instruction in regard to those functions and having been assessed as competent;
5. Work in a collaborative and co-operative manner with other health care professionals and recognize and respect their particular contributions within the health care team;
6. Take account of the customs, values and spiritual beliefs of patients/clients;
7. Make known to an appropriate person or authority any conscientious objection which may be relevant to professional practice;
8. Avoid any abuse of the privileged relationship which exists with patients/clients and of the privileged access allowed to their property, residence or workplace;
9. Respect confidential information obtained in the course of professional practice and refrain from disclosing such information without the consent of the patient/client or a person entitled to act on his/her behalf, except where disclosure is required by law or by the order of a court or is necessary in the public interest;
10. Have regard to the environment of care and its physical, psychological and social effects on patients/client or a person entitled to act on his/her behalf, except where disclosure is required by law or by the order of a court or is necessary in the public interest;
11. Have regard to the workload of and the pressures on professional colleagues and subordinates and take appropriate action if these are seen to be such as to constitute abuse of the

individual practitioner and/or to jeopardize safe standards of practice;

12. In the context of the individual's own knowledge, experience, and sphere of authority assist peers and subordinates to develop professional competence in accordance with their needs;

13. Refuse to accept any gift, favour or hospitality which might be interpreted as seeking to exert undue influence to obtain preferential consideration;

14. Avoid the use of professional qualifications in the promotion of commercial products in order not to compromise the independence of professional judgement on which patients/ clients rely.'

> *Code of Professional Conduct for Nurses, Midwives and Health Visitors, UKCC, 2nd Edn, (1984).*

Parliament, through the Nurses, Midwives and Health Visitors Act (1979) has passed legislation which allows nurses to decide what is acceptable in nursing, the above Code being the acceptable laid down standard.

A further UKCC advisory document, *Exercising Accountability* (1980) gives a framework to assist Nurses, Midwives and Health Visitors to consider ethical aspects of professional practice. This document supplements the Code of Professional Conduct.

Nurses, of course, are also on public display 24 hours of the day, even when off duty, and professional misconduct may occur on duty. If misconduct does occur on duty then it will be recognizable by the Code of Professional Conduct. Misconduct may also occur off duty when an act may be considered as anti-social or even criminal. Such offences are automatically reported to the relevant National Boards and the evidence would be considered and where necessary action taken.

INTERNATIONAL CODE OF NURSING ETHICS

There is also an International Code of Nursing Ethics which was first established in 1953 and was rewritten and adopted in 1973 by the International Council of Nurses. The Code is as follows:

The fundamental responsibility of the nurse is fourfold:

- to promote health;
- to prevent illness;
- to restore health;
- to alleviate suffering.

The need for nursing is universal. Inherent in nursing is respect for life, dignity and rights of man. It is unrestricted by consideration of nationality, race, creed, colour, age, sex, politics or social status.

Nurses render health services to the individual, the family and the community and co-ordinate their services with those of related specialties.

Nurses and people

- The nurse's primary responsibility is to those people who require nursing care;
- The nurse holds in confidence personal information and uses judgement in sharing this information.

Nurses and practice

- The nurse carries personal responsibility for nursing practice and for maintaining competence by continual learning;
- The nurse maintains the highest standards of nursing care possible within the reality of the specific situation;
- The nurse uses judgement in relation to individual competence when accepting the delegating responsibilities;
- The nurse, when acting in a professional capacity, should at all times maintain standards of personal conduct that reflect credit upon the profession.

Nurses and society

- The nurse shares with other citizens the responsibility for initiating and supporting action to meet the health and social needs of the public.

Nurses and co-workers

- The nurse sustains a co-operative relationship with co-workers in nursing and other fields;

- The nurse takes appropriate action to safeguard the individual when his care is endangered by a co-worker or any other person.

Nurses and the profession

- The nurse plays the major role in determining and implementing desirable standards of nursing practice and nursing education;
- The nurse is active in developing a core of professional knowledge;
- The nurse, acting through the professional organization, participates in establishing and maintaining equitable social and economic working conditions in nursing;

International Code of Nursing Ethics,
International Council of Nurses, (1973).

THE NURSES, MIDWIVES AND HEALTH VISITORS ACT OF 1979

This Act established the United Kingdom Central Council for Nurses, Midwives and Health Visitors, and the four National Boards. On 1st July, 1983, the UKCC and the Boards replaced the nine statutory and training bodies which until then had been responsible for training, education and the professional conduct of Nurses, Midwives and Health Visitors. The UKCC:

1. Maintains the professional Register of Nurses, Midwives and Health Visitors;
2. Establishes and improves standards of education and training;
3. Improves standards of professional conduct in order to protect the public from unsafe practitioners.

What is the Professional Register?

The Act of 1979 required the UKCC to establish a Professional Register. All Nurses, Midwives and Health Visitors who are entitled to practice in the United Kingdom are entered on a single Register.

All Nurses, Midwives and Health Visitors who have successfully applied for Registration have been added to the Register and have been allocated a Personal Identification Number (PIN).

Each person's entry on the Register includes all of the person's qualifications approved by the UKCC and each person is sent a copy of their entry when changes are entered in order to ensure that the information recorded on the Register is correct.

Each Nurse, Midwife and Health Visitor has a responsibility to inform the UKCC of any change, for example in name or address.

The main purpose of the Register is to protect the public. Any person who wishes to enquire about the registration status and the entitlement of any Nurse, Midwife and Health Visitor to practice may contact the UKCC for this information.

The UKCC and the four National Boards are also required under the 1979 Act to establish and improve standards of training for Nurses, Midwives and Health Visitors.

How does the Council improve standards of professional conduct?

The UKCC has produced a Code of Professional Conduct (already given in full) which sets out the expected standard of conduct for Nurses, Midwives and Health Visitors.

The UKCC has formulated rules which determine the circumstances under which a person's name may be removed from the Register and the circumstances by which a name be restored to the Register.

The four National Boards each have an Investigating Committee to consider cases of alleged misconduct by Nurses, Midwives and Health Visitors. These Committees, unless they decide no action is necessary, refer cases to the UKCC's Professional Conduct Committee or Health Committee.

Any person, whether or not a fellow professional, may contact the UKCC or appropriate National Board if they feel the safety of the public is threatened by the actions of any Nurse, Midwife or Health Visitor.

FUTURE TRENDS

The present Government's philosophy for health care is care in the community with the greater throughput of patients into the community, and the phasing out of large mental hospitals and mental handicap institutions. The mentally ill will be returned to live in the community within small units or mental health centres. The mentally handicapped will be housed in Community Homes where skilled assessment and planned training will be undertaken in order to determine and develop the full potential of each person.

There are increasing demands placed upon the community and primary care services because the elderly are living longer.

The public are becoming more aware of a healthy life-style and more are seeking help with regard to health promotion and illness prevention.

The social pressures of redundancy, lack of employment opportunities, the single parent, and those in the community who are addicted to smoking, alcohol or drugs remain.

The role of the Practice Nurse has expanded:

- the Practice Nurse is becoming increasingly involved in preventative and anticipatory care and health promotion;
- more patients/clients are making primary contact with the Practice Nurse specifically seeking advice and management from the Nurse;
- the number and variety of procedures the Practice Nurse undertakes has expanded.

Project 2000

It is hoped that the proposals of Project 2000 will meet these changes. The proposals are:

1. There will be a new single level of Nurse, whose role will embrace much of the work of present Registered and Enrolled Nurses;
2. A new Specialist Practitioner will undertake particular roles in the Hospital and the Community. These helpers should undertake specific tasks to provide care but be supervised by qualified Nurses, Midwives and Health Visitors. The roles of some specialist practitioners will be focused in particular areas of practice; others will work in health promotion. Specialist Practitioners will be people who have considerable experience and will have completed additional education programmes;
3. All the care required cannot be given by qualified Nurses, Midwives and Health Visitors alone. Project 2000 proposes that

helpers should be recruited to support Nurses, Midwives and Health Visitors;

4. A new pattern of education and training will be introduced. This should consist of a common foundation programme to be taken by all nursing students and will run for two years, followed by a programme in either the care of the adult, the child, of persons with mental handicap or in mental health;

5. Students will be super-numerary throughout their three year preparation and receive non-means-tested grants. Because nursing is a practical profession, the courses will have a high practical content and students will have patient/client contact. Project 2000 proposes that 20% of the student's time will be allocated to service contribution;

6. Education and training should be improved with more favourable teacher student ratios, and facilities comparable to the better standards to be found in tertiary education. Stronger links will be developed with colleges and institutions of higher and further education;

7. Enrolled Nurse training will cease but opportunities will be available for those Enrolled Nurses who wish to convert to Registered status.

Where next for Practice Nurses?

In order to make changes in the future both a short-term and long-term strategy needs to be determined.

Post-basic education

The present English National Board Course, which on successful completion gives the student a Statement of Attendance, is the foundation for the future. Any developments need to be based on evaluation of past and present courses and from informed research.

Practice Nurses have an individual responsibility to maintain and improve professional knowledge and experience. Such knowledge, experience, and professional competence might be gained through continuing education or research.

Continuing education can be summarized by the following activities:

- Supporting Practice Nurse interest groups;
- Organizing practice meetings with the practice team and members of the Primary Health Care Team in order to discuss clinical issues and practice procedures and protocols;
- Setting up and organizing a practice library;
- Attending conferences;
- Attending study days;
- Taking refresher courses;
- Reading professional journals, books and papers.

Research (see Chapter 10) involves identifying within the practice those patients/clients potentially at risk and setting up a research framework to monitor these patients.

Across the country there are some 230 Practices involved in research with the Medical Research Council. Such projects include:

- Hypertension in the elderly and the prevention of cerebrovascular accident;
- Thrombosis prevention trial – a low dose warfarin and aspirin trial for those at risk of a coronary thrombosis.

Developments

The developments of note for the future of Practice Nurses are:

1. The Government's support of Practice Nurses and central funding for their training;
2. The Government's support in recognizing the need for continuing education of the Practice Nurse and the development of distance learning packages;
3. The appointment of Nurse Facilitators to help practices set up projects to prevent patients suffering a myocardial infarction or cerebrovascular accident.
4. The post of Practice Nurse Adviser is now being considered by Family Practitioner Committees – giving advice and support to Practice Nurses and at the same time liaising with professional and statutory bodies.

FURTHER READING

Nurses, Midwives and Health Visitors Act (1979) HMSO, London.
Altschul, A. (1983) Shout at the Minister, Nursing Mirror, 157, 14, 21.

Editorial (1986) *Nursing Times*, 82, 11, 7.
Alleqay, L. (1986) Conduct unbecoming, *Nursing Times*, 82, 11, 19–20.
Professional Misconduct (1987) *Nursing Times*, 29–33.

Useful addresses

United Kingdom Central Council for Nursing,
Midwifery and Health Visiting,
23 Portland Place,
London, W1N 3AF.
Telephone: 01 637 7181

The Nurses Welfare Service
01 222 1563/4

Birmingham Drugline and Alcohol-related problems
021 632 6364

Any questions about training courses and entry into training should be
referred to the National Boards:

English National Board for Nursing, Midwifery and Health Visiting,
Victory House,
170 Tottenham Court Road,
London, W1P 0HA.
Tel: 01 388 3131

National Board for Nursing,
Midwifery and Health Visiting for Scotland,
22 Queen Street,
Edinburgh, EH2 1JX.
Tel: 031 226 7371

Welsh National Board for Nursing,
Midwifery and Health Visiting,
Thirteenth Floor,
Pearl Assurance House,
Greyfriars Road,
Cardiff, CF1 3AG.
Tel: 0222 395535

The National Board for Nursing, Midwifery
and Health Visiting for Norhern Ireland,
RAC House,
79 Chichester Street,
Belfast, BT1 4JE.
Tel: 0232 238152

4

Administration of the practice

Management is a science. It is the application of common sense based on a specialized knowledge in order to achieve short-term and long-term aims and objectives and to make plans to meet these objectives. In addition it is an art incorporating the ability to make decisions, determine priorities and implement them while maintaining at all times a good working relationship between staff.

Management in general practice is complex and all members of the practice staff, including those staff attached to the practice, will be involved in the process. The key person in the day-to-day management of a practice is the Practice Manager or Administrator. It is the manager who has the central co-ordinating role between patients, doctors, attached staff, support staff and outside agencies.

The emphasis today is on promoting health, preventing ill health and providing a health care service which is accessible, affordable and acceptable. The emphasis on primary health care presents a challenge not only to those in a clinical capacity working in primary care, but also to those who are involved in managing the service.

Management in general practice includes:

- Practice personnel;
- Communication systems;
- Premises;
- Health and safety.

PRACTICE PERSONNEL

Practice personnel may comprise:

- Doctors;
- Practice Nurse;

- Practice Manager/Administrator;
- Receptionist;
- Medical Secretary;
- Office Clerk/Medical Records Clerk;
- Data Clerks;
- Voluntary Workers;
- Attached staff:
  - Health Visitors
  - District Nurses
  - Community Midwives
  - Community Psychiatric Nurses
- Other specialist staff who may be employed by the practice, health authority or local authority:
  - Physiotherapist
  - Social Worker
  - Councellor
  - Chiropodist
  - Dietitian
  - Continence Nurse
  - Stoma Care Nurse
  - Community Mental Handicap Teams
  - Nurses who have undergone specialist training to help patients who have had major breast surgery.

Practice Manager/Administrator

The Practice Manager/Administrator has a central role and he/she carries out his/her responsibilities by planning, organizing, motivating and evaluating.

The following are some of the tasks and responsibilities of the Practice Manager:

Patients

- Organize clinics;
- Ensure confidentiality;
- Know as many patients as possible;
- Be prepared to listen;
- Ensure efficient systems are operating within the practice, and deal with any problems that may arise.

Doctors

- Organize surgeries;
- Plan duty rotas;
- Arrange locum cover as necessary;
- Organize support staff;
- Ensure efficient system of communication.

Staff

- Advertise, interview, appoint and review;
- Arrange education programmes and on-going in-service training;
- Organize meetings;
- Organize duty rotas;
- Encourage;
- Review performance.

Other agencies: communicate and liaise with

- Attached staff;
- Location Nurse Manager;
- Sector Managers of District Health Authority;
- Local Authority, e.g. Social Services;
- Family Practitioner Committee;
- Hospitals;
- District Health Authority;
- Royal College of General Practitioners;
- Local Medical Committee;
- Ambulance Service;
- Police Service;
- Pharmacists;
- Community Agencies;
- Voluntary organizations.

Finance

- Keep accounts;
- Balance books;

- Deal with:
  EPC quarterly returns;
  item of service payments;
  salaries and wages;
  petty cash;
  liaise with bank, accountant;
- Pay bills;
- Monitor cash flow.

Procedures or practice protocols

- For the administration of repeat prescriptions;
- Maintain age-sex register;
- Keep Red Book (Statement of fees and allowances) up-dated;
- Open and circulate mail;
- Monitor message book.

Building and supplies

- Order supplies;
- Ensure stocks are in hand;
- Maintenance of equipment;
- Check security system regularly;
- Arrange housekeeping and cleaning;
- Deal with furniture and decoration;
- Update noticeboard;
- Organize maintenance and repairs.

Information

- Run communication systems for patients, staff and doctors;
- Prepare practice statistics;
- Produce practice newsletter.

The following personal qualities required by a Practice Manager were identified by a group of Practice Managers attending a Training Course for Practice Managers and senior staff, run by the Royal College of General Practitioners (Thames Valley faculty) in conjunction with the Oxford Regional Health Authority (1980):

Quality	Attributes
Adaptability	Responding to emergency but still keeping long-term plans in view
Accessibility	Being accessible both physically (not always in remote office) and psychologically (being receptive to others)
Diplomacy	Smoothing troubled waters
Discretion	Asking the right questions, but not too bluntly
Fairness but firmness	Not having favourites
Humour	Defusing tension
Patience	Realizing that change does not happen overnight
Persuasiveness	Being able to convince with reason
Self-awareness	Knowing what one does best and the limits of one's authority and ability
Tact	Not putting one's foot in it
Trust	Creating an atmosphere where others can be open, by being open oneself
Unflappability	Counting to ten, even when things are hectic. Doing several jobs simultaneously.

In general terms, the Practice Manager needs to be able to:

1. Achieve a delicate balance between all aspects of his/her role;
2. Co-ordinate both the medical work and the administrative work of the practice;
3. Initiate;
4. Evaluate;
5. Show tolerance, sensitivity and understanding towards patients and all practice staff.

RECRUITMENT OF A PRACTICE MANAGER

Job description

A job description records the tasks and duties expected by the employer from an employee. This documentation provides the means of reference for employer and employee and can help in understanding of roles amongst colleagues. The duties of each member of staff will vary from practice to practice. It might be valuable to ask those staff already in a post to help in the formulation of a job description for any new employee.

Having completed the job description, the type of person required to fill the vacancy needs to be specified under the following headings:

- Age;
- Experience;
- Special skills;
- Personal attributes.

Advertising

From the job description and job specification, an advertisement can be prepared and placed in the agreed advertising media, which could be any of the following:

- Job Centre;
- Local newspaper;
- Local shop windows;
- Free local paper;
- A local College of Further Education which runs specific courses for the training of Practice Managers, Medical Receptionists, and Doctor's Receptionists;
- Local Groups of Practice Managers;
- The Association for Practice Managers, Medical Secretaries and Receptionists;
- Agency.

The purpose of the advertisement is to attract the right person for the vacancy. The advertisement should be based on the job description and job specification, stating the hours of work required and requesting the names of two referees.

Selection of candidates

The Job Description, details of holiday entitlement, sick pay and an application form or a request for a curriculum vitae will be sent to the potential applicant.

Shortlisting may be needed if there is considerable response to the advertisement. Such shortlisting may take place from the returned completed application details, and two or more references may be taken up.

On initial selection candidates may fall into the category of most suitable; possibly suitable; or definitely not suitable.

An interview, with more than one interviewer, should be arranged at a convenient, non-hurried time. The setting should be relaxed and as informal as possible. An opportunity should be made to show the interviewee around the practice and to meet other members of the staff.

A proforma of available details about the candidate is helpful, including such information as:

- Name;
- Address;
- Past experience;
- Health record past and present;
- Holiday arrangements already made;
- Interests;
- Commitments;
- When free to start if appointed.

It can be very difficult to make a decision when more than one candidate appears to be suitable for the vacancy. To help in this selection process the use of Rodger's Seven Point Plan may assist the interviewers to be more objective:

1. Physical make-up;
2. Attainments;
3. General intelligence;
4. Special aptitudes;
5. Interests;
6. Disposition;
7. Circumstances.

Using the job specification and Rodger's Seven Point Plan it is possible to draw up a score card. This score card can list the essential qualities needed for the job and the desirable qualities for the job.

Each candidate can be compared on essential qualities and if this still leaves the decision open then selection can be based on the desirable qualities of the candidate. If selection cannot be made the decision should be taken to re-advertise.

All applicants should be notified of their success or if they are unsuccessful.

Contract of employment

A contract exists immediately the post is offered verbally. The employee is entitled to a written Contract of Employment if they work 16 hours or more per week, under the Employment Protection (Consolidation) Act 1978.

The contract should contain the following:

- Name of parties to be contracted;
- Title of the Post;
- Details of pay scales and incremental dates;
- Sick pay;
- Method of payment and date of payment;
- Place of work;
- Hours of work;
- Holidays and arrangements for public holidays;
- Length of notice;
- Grievance procedure;
- Health and safety at work under the Act of 1974;
- Wearing of uniform or name badge;
- What will lead to instant dismissal.

Employment legislation

The employment law is complex and is for the protection of the employer, employee and the public. The law states the rights and obligations of both employer and employee.

Further details can be obtained from:

British Medical Association,
BMA House,
Tavistock Square,
London, WC1H 9JB.

The Association of Medical Secretaries, Practice Administrators and Receptionists (AMSPAR),

Tavistock House South,
Tavistock Square,
London, WC1H 9LN.

The Association of Health Centre and
Practice Administrators (AHCPA),
Lord Lister Health Centre,
121 Wood Grange Road,
London, E7 0EP.

Training courses

National courses for training in practice management are available
from:

- The Association of Health Centre and Practice Administration;
- The Association of Medical Secretaries, Practice Administrators
  and Receptionists;
- The *Practice Receptionist Programme* – a learning experience
  for receptionists – is now available at some Colleges of Further
  Education.

In-service training can involve orientation programmes and
continuing education programmes. All staff in post need regular
performances review.

COMMUNICATION

Communication is a two-way process covering both the imparting
of information and the receiving of information. Communication
can be either verbal or non-verbal.

The following factors are necessary for effective communication
between the Practice Manager and other staff:

- sensitivity;
- ability to see things from other people's point of views;
- regular meetings with staff;
- accessibility;
- listening;
- efficient and agreed systems of communication for the everyday
  running of the practice which all understand and follow.

The various means available for communication within a practice
are given below.

Message systems

Message book

This should ideally be completed under all the following categories:

- Date;
- Time of message;
- Identity for whom the message has been taken;
- Who message is from;
- Address and telephone number if appropriate of the person telephoning;
- Text of message;
- Message signed by the person taking and passing on the message;
- Confirmation when the message has been passed on.

All the staff are responsible for seeing that their messages have all been dealt with at the end of their period of duty, when a staff member goes off duty and at the end of the day.

Memoranda

Many practices use message pads or memoranda for passing messages. The use of a standardized and agreed procedure of memoranda format will help develop a uniform system of communication within the practice. A suitable example is given below.

Practice Name
Address

To:
From:
Date:
Time:

Message:

Signed:

Practice meetings

It is invaluable for the morale and motivation of all members of staff within the practice to meet regularly so there can be a two-way flow of information, and each staff member feels committed to and involved in the practice.

Practice meetings need to be well planned and well prepared and run with efficiency so that as little time as possible is wasted.

The John Cleese educational film *Meetings bloody meetings* (Video Arts Ltd, Dumbarton House, 68 Oxford Street, London) detailed the five steps necessary for the effective running of a meeting.

1. Planning ahead – aims and objectives of the meeting;
2. Pre-notification – inform those who are coming to the meeting of the items to be discussed;
3. Preparation – the agenda should follow through logically. Time should be allocated to the subjects on the agenda;
4. Processing – discussion of each item needs some structure: this is the role of the chairperson;
5. Putting it on record – a clear summary of the outcome of the meeting.

Newsletter

This form of communication can be for patients of the practice and for staff members. It can cover such topics as:

- Information with regard to changes in the practice;
- Thank-you messages from patients;
- Information with regard to visitors, meetings or research to be undertaken;
- Details of new staff members;
- Holidays.

This kind of communication can help all those involved with the practice to feel part of the practice team.

Practice booklet

New patients need to be made especially welcome and some practices arrange for new patients to be seen by the Practice Manager.

This initial meeting not only provides the opportunity of welcoming the patient to the practice and explaining in detail how the practice runs, but also gives an opportunity for patients to raise any issues or questions they may have.

Most practices produce a booklet or printed handout which will give some information such as:

- Name and address of practice;
- Telephone numbers over a 24-hour period for:
  - Emergencies
  - General enquiries
  - Appointments;
- Names of Doctors and staff;
- Surgery times;
- General medical consultations and other special facilities and clinics which operate from within the practice.

Noticeboard

It may be helpful for members of the practice staff to meet as a planning team to make decisions on the format of the information to be displayed on the practice noticeboard. The team might include the Practice Manager, a representative Receptionist, Practice Nurse, Health Visitor and District Nurse with the Health Education Officer within the District being a resource person.

Patient participation group

The involvement of a representative group of patients, doctors, support and attached staff of the practice meeting regularly can be a means of providing a listening post in the community. It can also be the means of implementing systems which could be to the benefit of patients in particular and the practice as a whole. Such systems might include:

- running a prescription collection service;
- operating a surgery car service;
- offering a good neighbour service to the ill, housebound and lonely;
- contributing to the practice newsletter.

THE PREMISES

The Doctor's Charter of 1966 allowed for the refunding of rent and rates and 70% reimbursement of staff salaries. Each Doctor will be refunded up to two whole time equivalents. This has resulted in many doctors in practice modernizing and extending their facilities.

The Statement of Fees and Allowances (Department of Health Guide) state that whilst doctors contract to provide medical services to their patients at the same time they also contract to provide adequate facilities for the patients within the practice.

Family Practitioner Committees are now required to visit general practice premises regularly. The aim of these visits is to assess the full range of facilities provided by a practice.

Design of new buildings

The Harding-Frast Report (DHSS, 1981a) recommended the following:

1. Eventual users of primary health care premises should be consulted during the initial design stages of the premises and be represented on the project team;
2. All new or adapted practice premises should be of sufficient size to accommodate the members of the team and their anticipated activities;
3. New or adapted premises should be designed, whenever possible, to facilitate informal contact between team members;
4. Any revision of the building note on health centres should take account of the comments in respect of size and design of facilities that should be provided that it should so far as possible be sufficiently broadly based to provide guidance on the design of group practice premises.

Much has been written about the design of doctor's surgeries and health centres, and the following information is available:

Design Guide for Medical GP Practice Centres,
Royal College of General Practitioners,
14, Princes Gate,
London, SW7 1PU.

Buildings for General Medical Practice,
HMSO, London.

Health Centres – a Design Guide,
HMSO, London.

When designing a new building the following factors need to be considered:

- Physical environment
  - lighting*;
  - ventilation*;
  - heating*;
  - sound control*;
  - fire exits and precautions. Any proposed new plans for a building have to meet the fire authority regulations. On request a fire officer will visit the practice and advise on any precautionary measures that need to be taken. Each practice should work out its fire plan carefully. It may be wise to arrange for a fire officer to meet the staff of the practice to explain fire drill*.
  - security – the crime prevention officers have undergone special training for their profession, their advice is free, and contact can be made through the local police station*;
  - safety features*.
- Psychological environment
  - pleasing colour schemes;
  - comfortable surroundings and chairs to sit in;
  - privacy for patients and staff;
  - plants, pictures, and up-to-date magazines all give the air of attention to individual comfort.

---

* from the 1st April, 1989 new fire precaution laws are operational. The Home Office have issued an advisory leaflet for Employers which states the circumstances in which a Fire Certificate is required and the circumstances when a Fire Certificate is not required.
  Details of detailed publication on the above are:
  Guide to fire precautions in places of work that require a fire certificate, HMSO, ISBN 113409060.
  Code of Practice for fire precautions in factories, offices, shops and railway premises not required to have a fire certificate. HMSO, ISBN 1134090044.
  A new guide which offers a basic but detailed information to employers, owners of businesses and for all who manage staff: Fire Safety at Work, HMSO, ISBN 113409052.

Maintenance

In order to present a welcoming atmosphere it is essential that the practice is maintained to a high standard.

The routine daily cleaning of the practice can be written down in the form of a work schedule. The Domestic will then have a cleaning programme to follow.

It may be necessary to employ a firm of cleaners to do the cleaning of the surgery on a regular basis to ensure reliability.

A weekly and monthly routine need to be planned and also a spring cleaning session bearing in mind that walls need to be washed and curtains cleaned.

The practice needs to be inspected regularly. All staff members should be encouraged to report any problems as soon as they are seen.

It is possible by regular inspection to note the necessary repairs, general maintenance and parts needing redecorating so areas of priority can be determined and an appropriate programme put into operation.

Redecoration of the practice on a rotational basis prevents a substantial financial outlay after years of no decoration.

HEALTH AND SAFETY

The Health and Safety at Work Act, 1974 is principally based on the report of the Robens Committee. This committee was set up to look at the health and safety of people whilst at work.

The 1974 Act applies to employment in general and not to any specific type of employment. The aim of the Act is to secure the safety, health and welfare of those persons at work and to protect those persons not at work from risks arising from the activities of those at work.

Duties of employers are statutorily laid down and obligations for the preparation of a policy statement with regard to health and safety which has to be produced in consultation with employee representatives is included in this statutory requirement of the Act.

Employees also have duties imposed upon them whereby they have duties to take due care of themselves and others with whom they may work.

The Act established the Health and Safety Commission which is responsible for producing legislation, codes of practice and safety guidelines relating to health and safety at work. This Commission is responsible to the Secretary of State.

The Health and Safety Executive is responsible for administering the Act on behalf of the Health and Safety Commission. They are an inspectorate group and have wide-ranging powers.

Duties of employers

Section 2.1 of the Act states: 'It shall be the duty of every employer to ensure, so far as is reasonably practicable the health, safety and welfare at work of all his/her employees'.

An employer is by law responsible for taking what reasonable measures are practicable to protect his/her workforce.

Section 2.2a '... the provision and maintenance of plant and systems of work that are, so far as is reasonably practicable, safe and without risk to health'.

Plant also includes equipment, machinery and appliances which are essential for the work undertaken; the appropriate equipment should always be provided and regularly maintained. A safe system of work is where all the known hazards have been considered and action taken to ensure there are no risks.

Section 2.2b '... arrangements for ensuring, so far as is reasonably practicable, safety and the absence of risks to health in connection with the use, handling, storage and transportation of articles and substances'.

This section is particularly appropriate when considering the handling of specimens, soiled dressings and such potential hazards as 'sharps' and is therefore of particular relevance to the Practice Nurse.

Section 2.2c '... the provision of such information, instruction, training and supervision as is necessary to ensure, so far as is reasonably practicable, the health and safety at work of his employees'.

No longer are employees expected to learn on the job. It is a requirement of the Act that employees are properly instructed and the potential hazards associated with any article, substance or piece of equipment are pointed out. It is also a requirement of the Act that proper supervision is given.

Section 2.2d '... so far as is reasonably practicable as regards any place of work under the employer's control, the maintenance of it in a condition that is safe and without risks to health and the provision and maintenance of means of access to and exit from it that are safe and without such risk'.

This section of the Act requires every place of work to be free from hazards which could be a potential risk to an employee.

Section 2.2e '... the provision and maintenance of a working environment for his/her employees that is, as is reasonably practicable, safe without risks to health and adequate as regards facilities and arrangements for their welfare at work'.

The atmosphere in which employees work should be free from risks. The lighting, heating, ventilation, seating, washing, toilet and eating facilities should all conform to legislation.

There are also duties laid down in the Act upon employers to ensure that those persons other than employees who visit the work place be it postman, milkman or others should not be put at risk in any way when visiting the premises.

Section 2.3 'Except in such cases as may be prescribed it shall be the duty of every employer to prepare and as often as may be appropriate revise a written statement of his/her general policy with respect to the health and safety at work of his employees and the organization and arrangements for the time being in force for carrying out that policy and to bring the statement and any revision of it to the notice of all his employees'.

If there are five or more employees there is a legal obligation on the part of the employer to produce a **safety policy**. The safety policy has three sections to it:

1. A statement of intent. This should state the employer's commitment to the safety and health of his/her employees and his/her intention to comply with legislation;
2. The organization and arrangements to put that statement into operation – or who does what. This will include written procedures and local arrangements designed to ensure the safety of all employees. It should also include the names of those who will take control in the event of any emergency;
3. The need to bring to the notice of all employees the points above including any revision. It is not sufficient to place the

safety policy on a noticeboard hoping that everyone will read it. An employer has a duty to ensure all employees have read and understood the safety policy.

Duties of employees

Under Sections 7 and 8 of the Health and Safety at Work Act, 1974 specific duties are placed upon the employee whilst at work, as follows.

Section 7.a '... to take reasonable care for the health and safety of himself/herself and of other persons who may be affected by his/her acts or omissions at work'

Employees have a duty to ensure that in their work and working environment they are not put at risk. An employee aware of a hazard has a duty to report it.

Section 7.b '... as regards any duty or requirement imposed on his/her employer or any other person by or under any of the relevant statutory provisions, to co-operate with him/her so far as is necessary to enable that duty or requirement to be performed or complied with'.

The employees have by law to co-operate to ensure the employer can meet his/her legal obligations.

Section 8 'No person shall intentionally or recklessly interfere with or misuse anything provided in the interests of health, safety or welfare in pursuance of any of the relevant statutory provisions'.

There is a legal obligation placed upon everybody not to interfere, misuse or damage anything that is provided as a statutory requirement. This would include fire extinguishers being used as door stops, fire doors being left open or exits being blocked.

Powers of Inspectors

Under the Health and Safety at Work Act, 1974 the Health and Safety Executive were given powers to appoint Inspectors to administer the law. The powers of Inspectors are as follows:

1. To enter premises at any reasonable time (normally when work is in progress);

2. To take a Police Constable on the visit if there is any reason to believe that the Inspector will be obstructed in the course of his/her duties;
3. To take with him/her any other person, that is an expert, and any other equipment necessary to assist in the inspection;
4. To make examinations and inspections;
5. To direct premises and equipment to remain untouched;
6. To take measurements, photographs and samples for analysis;
7. To take possession of any article or equipment for as long as necessary;
8. To examine books and documents and to take copies of same;
9. To require any person whom he believes has information to answer questions and to sign a declaration of the truth of the answers;
10. To dismantle destroy or make harmless any article or substance which in his/her opinion will cause imminent danger to health and safety.

If an Inspector is of the opinion that there has been or there is a breach of the statutory duty he/she will issue an improvement notice. This notice requires this breach to be rectified. The employer has the right of appeal within a 21-day period.

The Inspector may serve a prohibition notice if, in the opinion of the Inspector, there is a risk of serious personal injury. This notice can be served on a person or a piece of equipment. When a prohibition notice is served the relevant activities must cease. The employer has the right of appeal to an Industrial Tribunal.

Offences and penalties

Sections 33 and 37 outline the provisions concerning offences under the Health and Safety at Work Act, 1974. It is an offence for a person:

1. To fail to comply with any Section of the Act which imposes a duty;
2. To contravene any other health and safety regulation;
3. To contravene any requirement imposed by an Inspector;
4. To prevent any person from appearing before an Inspector to answer any questions or intentionally obstruct an Inspector in the course of his/her duties;

5. To contravene the requirements imposed by an improvement and prohibition notice;
6. To make a false statement or false entry in a register, book, notice or other document required under any statutory provision;
7. To deceive by forgery of a document;
8. To pretend to be an Inspector;
9. Not to comply with a Court Order.

Section 37 is concerned with offences by companies or partnerships and states:

> 'Where an offence under any of the relevant statutory provisions committed by a body corporate is proved to have been committed with the consent or connivance of or to have been attributable to any neglect on the part of, any Director, Manager, Secretary (Company) or other similar officer of the body corporate or a person who was purporting to act in any such capacity he as well as the body corporate shall be guilty of that offence and shall be liable to be proceeded against and punished accordingly'.

The liability for an act of neglect can be placed upon any person within a company or business setting. All persons need to observe and follow vigorously their responsibilities. Penalties can be applied to a company, an individual and/or a number of individuals.

Penalty may be in the form of a fine or imprisonment.

Accident prevention

The general responsibility for preventing accidents occuring rests with each individual. Every person should be conscious of safety. The following is a checklist:

- any person undertaking a specific task may see hazards others cannot; use this person's expertise in accident prevention planning;
- New employees by law must be supervised;
- Any staff member showing signs of being unwell should not continue to work;
- Special attention should be paid to walkways, floor coverings, and how premises are cleaned;

- All wounds, however small, should be treated appropriately and the accident book completed straight away;
- Daily inspection of the premises and equipment is essential: this provides a regular check on possible hazard areas.

Once a hazard has been identified the following action should be taken:

1. *Eliminate* remove the hazard if possible;
2. *Reduce or substitute* replace the hazard;
3. *Isolate* place a barrier between the hazard and personnel;
4. *Personal protection* it may be necessary to provide personal protection;
5. *Discipline* disciplinary procedure may be taken if safety legislation is not acted upon.

In conclusion, the Health and Safety at Work Act, 1974 aims at ensuring and safeguarding the health, safety and welfare of people. It places duties on everybody.

FURTHER READING

Employment of staff and employed staff

ACAS (Advisory Conciliation and Arbitration Service),
Clifton House,
Euston Road,
London, NW1 2RS.

British Institute of Management
Publication Sales,
Management House,
Parker Street,
London, WC2B 5PT.

The above Institute can provide checklists on such topics as:
- Staff vacancies
- Staff selection

British Medical Association,
BMA House,
Tavistock Square,
London, WC1H 9PJ.

Cullina, A., and Ellis, N., (1982) *Law and the General Practitioner.* Health and Safety at Work Act (1974).
Three articles in the *British Medical Journal* (1982) 285, pp. 1323, 1397, 1467.

These articles are available in booklet form from:
British Medical Association,
BMA House,
Tavistock Square.
London, WC1H 9PJ.

Ellis, N., (1981) *Pitfalls in Practice – Employment Law*
Ellis, N., (1983) *Law and the General Practitioner – Statutory Sick Pay*

Both the above publications are available in booklet form from:
British Medical Association,
BMA House,
Tavistock Square,
London, WC1H 9PJ.

The Seven Point Plan, by (the late) Professor Alec Rodger.
Paper No 1 3rd Edition (1970)
NFER – NELSON Publishing, Windsor, Berks.
Sidney, E., Brown, M., Argyle, M., (1973) *Skills with People*, Hutchinson, London.

Management of family practitioner services

Parr, C.W., Williams, J.P. (1981) *Family Practitioner Services and their Administration.*

The above publication is available from:
Institute of Health Service Administrators,
75 Portland Place,
London, W1N 4AN.

Pritchard, P.M.M., (1981) *Manual of Primary Health Care* (2nd Edn) Oxford University Press, Oxford.

Practice management

Jones, R.V.H., Bolden, K.J., Pereira Gray, D.J., and Hall, M.S., (1985) *Running a Practice: a Manual of Practice Management*, Croom Helm, London.
Metcalfe, D., (1982) *Information Systems and General Practice*, Pergamon Press, Oxford.

The Industrial Society,
Publications Department,
London, SW1Y 5BR.

The above Society has a comprehensive series of booklets for Managers, including such topics as:
Guide to employment practices
The Manager's guide to target setting
Guide to using the telephone
Motivation.

Design of new buildings

Department of Health Bibliography series HB 63 (surgeries) and HB 65 (Health Centres).
Obtainable from:
Department of Health
Health Building Library,
Room 1312, 286 Euston Road,
London, NW1 3DN.

Management in general

Drucker, P., (1974) *Management*, Heinemann, London.
Stewart, R., (1979) *The Reality of Management*, Pan Books, London.

Sources for obtaining audio-visual aid material:
Health Education Authority,
78 New Oxford Street,
London, WC1A 1AH.

Graves Medical Audio-Visual Library,
Holly House,
220 New London Road,
Chelmsford,
Essex, CM2 9BJ.

British Medical Association Film Library,
BMA House,
Tavistock Square,
London, WC1H 9JP.

Video-Arts Ltd.,
Dumbarton House,
68 Oxford Street,
London, W1N 9LA.

Pharmaceutical companies

Many pharmaceutical companies have a variety of video films available for
viewing in the practice/health centre setting.

Central Information Service for General Medical Practice,
14 Princes Gate,
London, SW7 1PU.

Health Services Management Centre,
University of Birmingham,
Park House,
40 Edgbaston Road,
Birmingham, B15 2RT.

King's Fund Centre Library,
126 Albert Street,
London, NW1 7NF.

Royal College of General Practitioners,
14 Princes Gate
London SW7 1PU

Royal College of Nursing,
20 Cavendish Square,
London, W1M 0AB.

5

The treatment room

Purpose-built surgeries should have treatment rooms and if this is not the case, the Practice Nurse should be involved in the planning of the treatment room. It may be helpful to visit operational treatment rooms in other practices or health centres before initiating plans.

The treatment room might be used for the following:

- Nursing procedures;
- Nursing treatments;
- Investigations;
- Examination;
- Specimen collection;
- Emergency treatments;
- Minor operations.

The Department of Health recommends a minimum size of 9.5 m² for the treatment room. The Department of Health has information with regard to design should this need to be referred to.

The treatment room has four main functions:

1. The treatment room itself should allow for minor operations, treatments and other procedures;
2. Storage area;
3. Preparation area;
4. Space where the doctor, nurse and patients can consult.

DESIGN

The design of the treatment room should include the following features:

- Privacy;
- Ease of access and exit (following fire regulations);
- All surfaces should be washable and easy to clean;
- The Treatment Room should be straightforward to maintain;
- Well ventilated;
- Well heated;
- Bright and pleasing to the eye;
- Working space for the nurse not only for treatment but for paperwork and talking to patients;
- Easy access and means of communication for staff and patients;
- Adequate electrical power points;
- A separate waiting area associated with the Treatment Room for those patients waiting to see the nurse;
- Flooring which is non-slip and easy to clean and maintain.

EQUIPMENT

Treatment room equipment will be the responsibility of the Practice Nurse and will include:

- refrigerator for storage of vaccines (refrigerator should have a thermometer guage so vaccines can be stored at appropriate temperature);
- furniture;
- linen including blankets, pillows, paper sheets and towels;
- a range of sterile dressings and surgical packs;
- plaster of Paris;
- selection of splints;
- lotions;
- suturing materials;
- instruments;
- specialized equipment.

The following lists give detailed requirements for equipment under the appropriate headings.

Equipment for general nursing procedures

Furniture

- Trolley;
- Couch;

- Light(s);
- Scales – baby, adult;
- Height measure;
- Length measure for babies.

Surgical equipment

- Nebulizer;
- Auroscope;
- Ear syringing equipment;
- Nasal speculum;
- Spatulae;
- Stethoscope;
- Sphygmomanometer;
- Tourniquet;
- Vaginal speculae;
- Sonic-aid and/or fetal stethoscope;
- Latex disposable gloves;
- Sharps container;
- Torch;
- Mirror;
- Container for liquid nitrogen;
- Transformer and leads for cautery;
- Sight testing – Keeler.

Other equipment for use by Doctor using treatment room

- Ophthalmoscope;
- Proctoscope;
- Handle and Eyes for cautery procedures;
- Percussors;
- Tuning Forks.

Other instruments

- Scissors – all types and sizes;
- Spencer Wells artery forceps;
- Dissecting forceps;
- Tooth dissecting forceps;
- Tissues holding forceps;

- Bard Parker holder and blades;
- Stitch cutters;
- Clip removers;
- Needle holder(s);
- Curettes.

Equipment for IUCD fitting and IUCD checks

- Scissors;
- Sponge-holding forceps;
- Vulsellom;
- Uterine sound;
- Spencer Wells forceps;
- Cusco's speculum.

Equipment for suturing

- Needle holder;
- Suture material;
- Scissors;
- Tooth dissecting forceps;
- Spencer Wells forceps.

Investigative equipment

- Electrocardiograph;
- Peak flow meter;
- Centrifuge;
- Blood sugar meter;
- Urine testing equipment;
- Specimen containers;
- Needles, syringes and swabs and transport medium;
- Haemoglobinometer;
- Auto-meter for measuring cholesterol levels;
- Auto-analyser for a variety of blood tests.

EMERGENCY TRAYS

All practices should have the means to resuscitate patients in the event of collapse and have the means immediately available to deal with lacerations and wounds resulting from an injury. Trays should also be ready for dealing with foreign bodies in the eye and for immobilizing a suspected fracture. The contents of the various trays are listed below.

Collapse tray

- Airways;
- Mouth gag;
- Tongue forceps;
- Injection Hydrocortisone 100 mg for IV or IM injection;
- Injection Aminophyline 250 mg in 10 ml;
- Injection Dextrose 50% in 25 ml for IV use;
- Injection Adrenaline 1/1000 in 1 ml for IM use;
- Injection Prochlorperazine 12.5 mg in 1 ml;
- Injection Atropine Sulphate 600 in 1 ml;
- Injection Terbutaline 0.5 mg in 1 ml;
- Injection Diazepam 10 mg in 2 ml;
- Injection Frusemide 20 mg in 2 ml;
- Injection Salbutamol 0.5 mg in 1 ml;
- Tablets Chlorpheniramine 4 mg;
- Tablets Diazepam 2 mg in 5 mg;
- Shock blanket;
- Emergency delivery pack;
- 'Spill-Pak' for blood, urine and other body fluids;
- Giving-sets.

The Modulaide Doctor Emergency Case produced by Laerdal is equipped for: ventilation; suction; intubation; infusion; injection; and wound treatment.

Laryngeal tray

- Xylocaine throat spray;
- Laryngeal mirror;
- Head mirror and strap;
- Methylated spirit lamp and matches;
- Nasal forceps;
- Long throat forceps;
- Tongue spatulae;
- Swabs.

Eye tray

Sterile minimsol:
- Fluorescein 1%;
- Sodium Chloride 0.9%;
- Chloramphenicol;
- Amethocaine 1%;
- Mydrilate 0.5%;
- Atropine Sulphate 1%;
- Eye pads and tape.

Suture tray

- Dressing pack (sterile);
- Cleaning agent;
- Sterile needles and syringes;
- Local anaesthetic – Lignocaine 1% plain;
- Assorted sizes of steri-strips;
- Assorted atraumatic cutting needles and silk;
- Nobecutane plastic wound dressing spray.

STOCK CONTROL – ORDERING AND MAINTENANCE

Equipment

Each piece of equipment should be entered as an item in Stock Control, giving its date of purchase and regular maintenance interval as well as the basic method of routine cleaning after use.

Lotions

Basic lotions should be stored and the quantity needs to be entered in a Stock Control filing system and ordered monthly as appropriate, or according to shelf life.

Medication

A monthly check needs to be make on all stock to ensure no drugs are outside their recommended date of use. In addition the relevant stock needs to be kept up-dated using a local pharmacist for regular ordering. Controlled drugs will be entered in the Drug Book and reviewed from time to time by the Regional Medical Officer. Storage of controlled drugs and any medication must follow the standard regulations.

Records

In order to maintain stock levels and to ensure equipment is regularly maintained, use should be made of the practice computer; card filing systems; and a diary.

6

Nursing models

The Nursing Models described in this Chapter are ones developed by Roper and Roy. Roper's model has been adopted to have the nursing process incorporated within it.

A Nursing Model is based on a model of living. Most members of the public only require nursing intervention episodically during their lives and the rationale of linking nursing with living was that there should be minimal interruption of a client's usual way of living whilst he/she needed nursing intervention. Maslow's hierarchy of needs may help the nurse to set priorities when nursing intervention for a client is indicated.

The focus of the model is on the individual's activities of living:

1. Maintaining a safe environment;
2. Communicating;
3. Breathing;
4. Eating and drinking;
5. Eliminating;
6. Personal cleansing, hygiene and dressing;
7. Controlling body temperature;
8. Mobilizing;
9. Working and playing;
10. Expressing sexuality;
11. Sleeping;
12. Dying.

The activities of living used in conjunction with the nursing process provide the framework for assessment, planning, implementation and evaluation which make up the stages of the process.

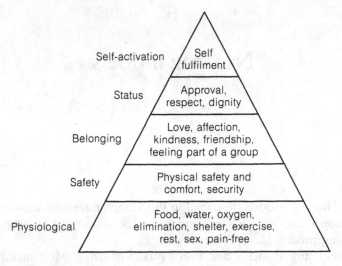

Figure 6.1 Maslow's Hierarchy of Needs can help the nurse to set priorities.

Because the model focuses on living, it encourages the patient/ client to be central to the model.

The emphasis on activities of living also encourages an emphasis on health promotion and prevention of ill health, as well as the care of the unwell person.

Roy's Systems Model looks at an individual on a health/illness continuum which is influenced by the person's ability to adapt to stimuli – focal, contextual and residual. The aim of nursing is to help that individual to adapt to stimuli on one or more of four adaptive modes:

1. Physiological needs;
2. Self-concept;
3. Role function;
4. Interdependence.

Roy's Adaptation Model focuses on the individual, but the recipient of nursing may be an individual, a family, a group, a community and/or society. Such an adaptive system involves input, internal and feedback processes and output. The individual is seen as a biopsychosocial being who is in constant interaction with his/ her internal and external environment. Nursing in this context helps the individual by promoting and supporting his/her adaptive abilities.

THE PATIENT – THE NURSING PROCESS; A WAY TO BETTER HEALTH

The Nursing Process appeared on the scene in Britain in the early 1970s. The process is basically the problem-solving approach applied to nursing.

Table 6.1 *Components of the nursing process compared to components of problem solving*

Nursing process	Problem solving
Assessment	
Collect data – Nursing	Recognize and define the
Clarify the data	problem
Analyse the data	
Summarize the data	
Problem identification	
Interpret the data, through critical analysis	
Male nursing diagnosis through statement of the problem	
Planning nursing intervention	
Devise nursing care plan	Formulate the plan
State objective	
State criterion for evaluation to measure objective	
List nursing alternatives that could meet the objective	
Implementation	
Communicate plan to team	Implement the plan
Coordinate patient care	
Evaluation	
Examine patient behaviour in relation to evaluation criterior	Evaluate the plan

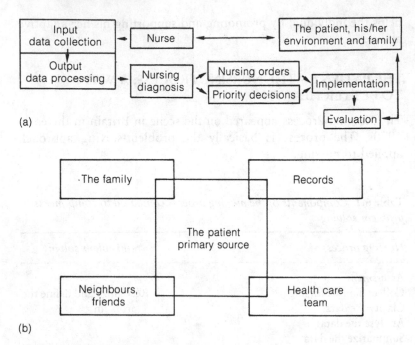

(a)

(b)

Figure 6.2 The nursing process in action — continuous feedback (a); resources for patient assessment (b).

This process is made up of four stages:

1. Assessment – The collection from any available source particularly the patient or client of information which is relevant to his/her health state and care.

   The end of this stage is the identification of nursing problems, patient problems or nursing diagnosis. It should be a succinct statement of the indications for nursing action;

2. Planning – Objectives, goals or desired outcomes are set and plans made to work towards achieving them. These indicate what the patient/client will be able to do and what his/her condition will be if the plan is successful;

3. Implementation – The plan is put into action;

4. Evaluation – In this stage a check is made to see whether the care given seems to have been wholly or partially successful in achieving the desired outcome.

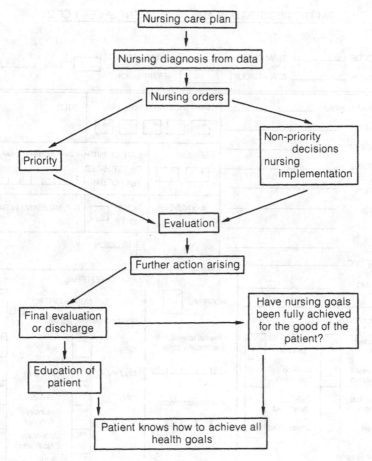

Figure 6.3 Flow chart of a nursing care plan.

All the stages focus on aspects of individual nursing care. In practice the four stages cannot be neatly separated since one or more of the stages may be occurring at the same time.

Essential features of the Nursing Process are that as far as possible the patient/client should participate in each stage and, where relevant, the patient/client's family and friends should be involved.

The following diary sheets used for patient registration and assessment provide the means of implementing a framework for nursing (these diary sheets are used in Bromley Health District).

PATIENT REGISTRATION AND ASSESSMENT SHEET 1 OF 2

STAFF CODE └──────┘   TEAM CODE └──────┘   AMENDMENT TO ▢   DATE └─/─/─┘

STAFF NAME ─────────   STAFF GROUP ▭   REGISTRATION

PATIENT NUMBER ─────────────

SURNAME ─────────────

FORENAME ─────────────

ADDRESS ─────────────

─────────────

─────────────

─────────────

POST CODE ─────────────

TEL. NO. ─────────────

MARITAL STATUS (tick)

| M | S | W | D | Sep |

TITLE

SEX (tick)

| M | F |

DATE OF BIRTH   DAY   MONTH   YEAR
OR ESTIMATED
YEAR OF BIRTH └─┴─┴─┴─┴─┴─┘

NHS NUMBER

TICK IF ▢ NO G.P.

G.P. NAME AND INITIALS

RELIGION

EMPLOYMENT (tick):

Long term sick	A	Working full-time	E
Housewife/ Husband	B	Working part-time	F
Student/at School	C	Self-employed	G
Retired	D	Unemployed	H

Other (specify)

SOURCE OF REFERRAL

HOSPITAL ▢ H

NON-HOSPITAL ▢ NH

Hospital referral give hospital code

└ H ┴─┴─┴─┴─┘

and specialty code

└─┴─┴─┴─┘

Non-hospital referral (tick):

GP	NH1	Self	NH9
DN / HV	NH2	Local Authority	NH10
CPN	NH3	Social Services	NH11
CMHN	NH4	Voluntary Services	NH12
MO	NH5	Ante-Natal Notification	NH13
Midwife	NH6	Birth Notification	NH14
Education	NH7	Other (specify):	
Relative	NH8		

NEXT OF KIN:	CONTACT PERSON:	PRINCIPLE DIAGNOSIS:
SURNAME _____	SURNAME _____	
FORENAME _____	FORENAME _____	TREATMENT REQUIRED/ PURPOSE OF VISIT
ADDRESS _____	ADDRESS _____	
_____	_____	CHIEF CARER:
TEL NO. _____	TEL NO. _____	RELATIONSHIP _____
RELATIONSHIP _____		Sex _____ Approx Age _____

OTHER PERSONAL DETAILS

SOLITUDE:

	0-2	2-10	10+		YES	NO
Hours alone by day	A	B	C	Alone at night	Y	N

OTHER AGENCIES (tick)

OT Social Services	A	CPN	F
Social Worker	B	CMHN	G
Voluntary Visiting Scheme	C	OT Hospital	H
Speech Therapy	D	HV/ON	J
Community Physiotherapist	E	School/Nurse	K

Other (specify)

BENEFITS RECEIVED (tick)

Attendance Allowance	A	Private Pension	D
Supplementary Benefit	B	Rent Rebate	E
Mobility allowance	C	Rate Rebate	F

Other (specify)

REFERRED TO (tick)

FURTHER HEALTH CARE

G.P.	RA1	OT Hospital	RA8
MO	RA2	OT Soc Services	RA9
HV (including specialist HV)	RA3	Physiotherapist	RA10
CPN	RA4	Hospice	RA11
CMHN	RA5	Marie Curie	RA12
Speech Therapy	RA6	Eve Nursing service	RA13
Chiropody	RA7	Night Sitting service	RA14

Other (specify)

OTHER AGENCIES

Social services	RB1
Education	RB2
Meals on wheels	RB3
Home help	RB4
Night watch	RB5
Voluntary visiting	RB6

Other (specify)

SOCIAL SUPPORT (tick)

Lives alone	A	Lives with other relatives	E
Lives with spouse	B	Lives with children only	F
Lives with spouse and adult children	C	Lives with parents	G
Lives with brothers/sisters	D	Other (specify)	

REGULAR HELP (tick)

	M	T	W	Th	F	Sc	Sn	Less than (per week)	PRN
	A	B	C	D	E	F	G	H	J
Relations/ Neighbours	0								
Wardens	1								
Meals on wheels	2								
Home help/ Community Care	3								
Day Hospital	4								
Day Centre	5								
Night Watch	6								
Night Nurse	7								
Marie Curie	8								
Cross roads	9								

NURSING ASSESSMENT REQUIRED	YES	NO

PATIENT REGISTRATION AND ASSESSMENT SHEET 2 OF 2

DATE ⌊ / / ⌋ Patient Number _____ 1st Assessment ☐

STAFF CODE ⌊_____⌋ Patient Name _____ Reassessment ☐

STAFF NAME _____ Sex [M] [F] Date of Birth ⌊ / / ⌋ Amendment to Assessment ☐

MOBILITY	Without Help	With aid	Needs 1 Helper	Needs 2 Helpers	Not able
Walking	A	B	C	D	E
Climbing stairs	A	B	C	D	E
Rising from chair	A	B	C	D	E
In/out of bed	A	B	C	D	E
Dressing/Undressing	A	B	C	D	E
Use of WC/Commode	A	B	C	D	E
Getting out of the house	A	B	C	D	E

PERSONAL HYGIENE					
Washing hands/face	A	B	C	D	E
Shaving	A	B	C	D	E
Hair care	A	B	C	D	E
Bathing	A	B	C	D	E
Care of feet	A	B	C	D	E
Keeping clothes clean	A	B	C	D	E
Keeping room/house clean	A	B	C	D	E

FEEDING					
Feeding self	A	B	C	D	E
Preparing food	A	B	C	D	E
Fetching food	A	B	C	D	E

DIET

	YES	NO
Is diet satisfactory	☐	☐
If no, give details		

COMMUNICATION

Problems with: (specify any problem)

Talking

Hearing

Sight

Other

PAIN

Bowel Y/N [B]   Micturition Y/N [M]

None	Intermittent Mild	Intermittent Severe	Continual Mild	Continual Severe
A	B	C	D	E

MENTAL STATE

	No problem	Occasional problem	Severe problem
Orientation	A	B	C
Memory	A	B	C
Aggression	A	B	C
Anxiety	A	B	C
Depression	A	B	C
Confusion	A	B	C
Motivation	A	B	C
Sociability	A	B	C

BREATHING (tick)

		Breathless	C
Smoker	A	Cyanosed	D
Non-smoker	B	Oxygen	E

WARMTH

	YES	NO
Keeps warm If no, tick reason	Y	N

Inadequate clothing	A	Inadequate heating	C
Heating not used	B	Heating unavailable	D

BLADDER PROBLEMS (tick)

Catheter	A
Incontinence Night	B
Incontinence Day	C
Incontinence Stress	D
Urastomy	E

BOWEL PROBLEMS (tick)

Constipation	A
Incontinence	B
Stoma	C

HOUSING

House	A	Owner Occupied	A
Hotel/Room	B	Local Authority	B
Flat	C	Private rented	C
High Rise	D	L.A. Residential	D
Bungalow	E	Private Residential	E
Sheltered Accom	F	Other	F
Mobile Home	G		

URINE TEST

	Tick	Result			Tick	Result
Blood	A			Glucose	C	
Ketones	B			Protein	D	
				pH	E	

Stairs to entrance [ ] Y/N

Stairs to toilet [ ] Y/N

Is bed downstairs [ ] Y/N

FURTHER READING

Hunt, J., and Marks-Maron, D. (1980) *Nursing Care Plans*, MS and M, Aylesbury.

Maslow, A.H. (1970) *Motivation and Personality*, Harper and Row, London.

Orem, D.E. (1980) *Nursing: Concepts of Practice*, 2nd Edn, McGraw Hill, New York.

Roper, N., Logan, W.W., and Tierney, A.J. (1981) *Learning to use the Process of Nursing*, Churchill Livingstone, Edinburgh.

Roper, N., Logan, W.W. and Tierney, A.J. (eds) (1983) *Using a Model for Nursing*, Churchill Livingstone, Edinburgh.

Roy, C., and Roberts, S.L. (1971) *Theory Construction in Nursing: An Adaptation Model*, Prentice Hall, New Jersey.

7

Screening as a function of primary care

Major medical advances during the past century have been made in the field of prevention.

There remain diseases associated with people's life-style where concerted screening efforts should help to reduce mortality and morbidity rates. These diseases include:

- Coronary artery disease;
- Carcinoma of the lung;
- Bronchitis;
- Sexually transmitted disease including AIDS;
- Addiction.

The Government places emphasis on screening for health in its White Paper, *Promoting Better Health* (1987).

WHAT IS SCREENING?

Screening is the detection of disease before signs and symptoms appear.

Changes in the prevalence of disease have been brought about by:

1. Immunization programmes
2. Government education programmes, legislation and research, including:
   (a) Health hazard warnings on: smoking; alcohol; AIDS and sexually transmitted diseases.
   (b) Legislation on seat-belts and additives in food products.

(c)   Research into life-style; thrombosis prevention; hypertension in the elderly.
3.   Greater awareness by the public who recognize the need to change their life-style to avoid unpleasant consequences.

The purpose of screening is to: reduce morbidity; reduce mortality; and improve the quality of life.

Types of screening

Opportunistic

This is a haphazard approach. When the patient presents at the surgery to make an appointment, organize a repeat prescription request or to collect a prescription, or for consultation, he/she is either offered further health screening there and then or offered an appointment with the Practice Nurse for a health screening check.

Planned approach

This method identifies a group of patients whether by age, sex or medical problem to whom health screening will be offered.

Patients can be identified by: the age-sex register; by colour-coded records for medical conditions (The Royal College of General Practitioners provides guidelines on colour coding for tagging records and age-sex cards); and by computer, by running a disease index audit. Figure 7.1 shows examples of codes for age-sex cards and colour codes for patient's records.

There are currently Nurse Facilitators being appointed through Family Practitioner Committees to help practices set up screening programmes.

Before setting up a screening programme, the practice needs to decide:

● Priority groups to be screened;
● The best person(s) to undertake the screening;
● A formal protocol to follow;
● The most opportune time to undertake the screening programme;
● A place for screening – availability of consultation room/ nurse's consultation room;

(a) Age-sex card

A.S.R.2a   THE ROYAL COLLEGE OF GENERAL PRACTITIONERS

Dr. Code								Surname of Patient			Forename		Date of Birth				Sex	MS	SS
1	2	3	4	5	6	7	8	9	10	11	12		13–14	15–16	17–18	19	20	21

Addresses
1.

2.

3.

Occupation

N.H.S. No.

E.C.

Date (Entry) _____   22–33 | 24–25 | 26–27

Date (Removal) _____ 28–29 | 30–31 | 32–33

Reason _____   34 | 35

Card to E.C. / /19

A	B	C	D	E	F	G	H	I	J	K	L	M	N	O	P	Q	R	S	T	U	V	W	X	Y	Z
36	37	38	39	40	41	42	43	44	45	46	47	48	49	50	51	52	53	54	55	56	57	58	59	60	61

(b) Codes for age-sex card

Key to *Box*: 36   First triple and polio
            37   Second triple and polio
            38   Third triple and polio
            39   Measles/mumps/rubella (measles)
            40   Pre-school diptheria, tetanus and
                  polio or/and measles/mumps/rubella
            41   Rubella (if not in box 39)
            44   Cervical smear at age 35 years
            45   Cervical smear at age 40 years

(c) Colour codes for patients' records

Hypertension	blue
Diabetes	brown
Epilepsy	yellow
Sensitivities	red
Psychiatric illness	green
Long-term-medication	white
Attempted suicide	black

Figure 7.1 Examples of coding for patients' records (a) age–sex card;
(b) codes for age–sex card; (c) colour codes for patients' records.

- How to inform support and attached staff and plan and implement in-service training;
- What equipment, if any, needs to be purchased.

Having decided on the target group, the practice needs to determine how to identify the patients of the target group, whether opportunistically through: attendance at the surgery for any reason; coded records; age-sex register; or computer; or as a planned exercise through:

- Placing a notice on practice noticeboard inviting the patients in the target group to attend for screening;
- Publicizing the screening programme through the practice newsletter;
- Using a representative of the practice's consumer group to disseminate the information;
- Offering patients an appointment at their first visit to the practice;
- Sending a personal letter of invitation.

Aim of screening

The aim of screening is to determine the presence or absence of disease or disease risk factor(s) in an individual who had no apparent symptoms or signs of the disease.

Target groups for screening might be:

1. Special risk groups, such as
   (a) Those patients with a family history of hypertension or coronary heart disease
   (b) Obese patients
   (c) Hypertensive patients
   (d) Patients who smoke
   (e) Patients who suffer from diabetes mellitus;
2. New patients;
3. Children – development and surveillance;
4. Well Woman;
5. Well Man (MOT);
6. Elderly.

When screening new patients, the aims are:

- To identify any person new to the practice who may have an already known problem for whom regular follow-up needs to be established;
- To identify any person who may have an incipient problem and to refer for investigation/treatment;
- To identify those at risk;
- To record relevant medical and family history about the patient for future reference and if appropriate enter onto the computer;
- To record information such as:
  - immunization status
  - cervical cytology
  - smoking
  - alcohol habits;
- To establish a recall system;
- To establish relationships within the primary health care setting.

Screening procedure

Approximately 15 minutes should be allocated to each patient for the health check, and the reason for the interview and health check should be explained to the patient. The health check should consist of the following points:

- Record the patient's blood pressure;
- Measure and record the patient's height and weight;
- Test the urine;
- Give appropriate advice;
- Refer to the general practitioner;
- Arrange follow-up, if necessary.

Records of the results obtained from screening can be kept as a health summary (example in Figure 7.2) or in the form of a health questionnaire (Figure 7.3).

SCREENING THE ELDERLY

The present philosophy of care of the elderly is for them to remain in their own homes as long as possible with the support of their families, the primary health care services, social services and

Surname		Forenames		dob		sex M F

Address

Occupation	Partner's occupation

Medical History

Family Profile	Diabetes	HT	MI	CVA	Epilepsy	Asthma	Glaucoma	Death
Mother								
Father								
Siblings								
Children								

Obstetric History

Height	Ideal Weight

Year								
WT								
BP								
Urine								
Cx Smear								

Breasts Testicles	
Oral Cp.	
Tetanus	
Polio	
Rubella	
Alcohol	

Exercise

Notes/Advice given/follow-up

Figure 7.2 Health summary.

NAME
DATE OF BIRTH
OCCUPATION
ADDRESS

TELEPHONE NO.

Have you had any serious illnesses?   Please list

Have you had any operations?   Please list

Have you had any accidents?

Current medication if any:

Please list any allergies or reactions to medicine or vaccine

Immunization: are you protected against

*Tetanus   Date if known
*Polio

Have you ever smoked?	Yes	No
If Yes at what age did you start?	Age	
Do you still smoke	Yes	No
At what age did you stop?	Age	

If a smoker what is your consumption   .... cigarettes/day
                                                                   .... cigars/day
                                                                   .... ounces tobacco/day

How much alcohol do you drink?   Beer   ... pints/week
                                                            Wine   ... glasses/week
                                                            Spirits ... singles/week

FAMILY HISTORY				
DEAD	LIVING		DEAD	
	AGE	STATE OF HEALTH	AGE	CAUSE OF DEATH
FATHER				
MOTHER				
BROTHERS				
SISTERS				

Is there a family history of:

Heart disease	Yes	No
Diabetes	Yes	No
Raised blood pressure	Yes	No
Stroke	Yes	No
Asthma	Yes	No

Female patients – children please list:

Date of birth   Sex   Place of birth   Any difficulties with
pregnancy or birth

Have you had a cervical smear test?

Date of last cervical smear:

Have you been taught how to examine your breasts?   Yes   No

Are you taking oral contraceptives?   Yes   No

For how long?

Date of last check?

Are you using any other form of contraceptive, if Yes please state what form and when you were last checked

Form of contraceptive:

Date of last check:

Do you require help or advice with contraception?

Have you had a blood test to see if you are immune to Rubella (German Measles)?

Figure 7.3 Health questionnaire for new patients.

voluntary agencies such as Age Concern. The support needs to focus upon activity, stimulation, motivation, diet, warmth, and company.

Age alone, of course, is not a predictor of health status, but dependency upon others does increase in old age and very often symptoms of illness and/or social need are either left or remain undiagnosed until the patient has a major problem.

Screening the elderly provides a preventative, systematic and caring approach and whilst many patients appreciate this increased interest in them by the Primary Care Team, others resent the intrusion into their privacy and are content to stay the way they are.

The target population can be identified through:

- Practice profile statistics;
- Age-sex register;
- Computer;
- Elderly at risk register.

Methods of identifying the needs of patients for screening

Some base their screening programme within the practice health centre setting where immediate access to other facilities is available such as chiropody, social worker, and dentist.

Some use the pretext of offering an anti-flu injection as a means of access into the patient's home and use this time to assess the patient and home environment.

Others carry out the assessment in the home setting after informing the patient of the visit. The most readily acceptable person to do this assessment might be the Practice Nurse, who is specifically employed in some instances to undertake this role. Other practices employ a team approach, with the attached Health Visitor, District Nurse and Practice Nurse all sharing in the assessment.

Some practices send health questionnaires for completion; others use the questionnaire method but send it to their patients on their birthdays as a greetings card.

The team involved in screening the elderly

Each member of the team has an important role to play and needs to be aware of the whole programme and the part they individually play.

Close liaison with all those involved in providing help to the elderly is essential. Regular communication, possibly in the form of team meetings, can enhance relationships and may help to identify the need for a different approach to a particular patient's programme of care. Such communication also provides the opportunity to continuously assess the practice team's needs, the elderly patient population of the practice and their needs, and the practice protocol on screening and care of the elderly and their supporters.

Problems associated with the elderly

Apathy

Loneliness and loss of motivation can lead to forgetfulness and failure to care for themselves.

Anaemia

This condition may be due to possible iron deficiency because of poor diet. It may also arise from blood loss due to haemorrhoids which may have not been treated for sometime, or from aspirin ingestion over many years leading to gastro-intestinal bleeding. Other drug intake, such as anti-inflammatory medication, may also lead to anaemia.

Endocrine disorders

These may be caused by late onset diabetes or thyroid abnormalities.

Incontinence

Incontinence of urine is a common problem and is one where the cause should be investigated and the appropriate treatment instigated.

Incontinence of faeces similarly needs to be investigated and the patient helped in an appropriate way.

Senses

Many elderly patients need special help with hearing and vision.

Activity

A number of elderly suffer from musculo-skeletal diseases such as osteoarthritis, osteoporosis and experience muscle weakness and joint pain through lack of movement. The fact that they are less mobile or find it more difficult to bend or tend to fall more readily can lead to numerous problems, such as toe nails not being cut, long bone fractures, and hypothermia.

Hypothermia

Many elderly do not have a sufficiently warm environment or adequate diet. The elderly tend to sit still for a good part of the day. Very often they feel cold, don't change position and ultimately collapse. They may, of course, be unable to reach the switch of a plug at ground level or they may be worried because of the expense of keeping warm.

Confusion/forgetfulness

Lack of motivation, company and someone to talk to may mean the patient fails to take the medication prescribed, and a confused forgetful state puts the patient at risk of accidents in the home.

Social

Loneliness is often a problem in the elderly.

Social service benefits may not be applied for because of their complexity.

Fear of mugging and increasingly the fear of rape mean that many elderly persons are afraid to go out.

Gadgets and aids which are available may not be known to the elderly person who needs them.

The assessment

The home assessment of an older person provides crucial information on the patient's present state of health, and also gives indicators for future management. A change in the appearance of the patient's home may be an important pointer of the patient's inability to manage. The following points should be noted on a home visit.

Outdoors

- State of the garden;
- Upkeep of the house/flat.

At the door

- How long does it take the patient to answer the door?
- The state of the patient when the door is opened;
- How does the patient stand – is support needed?
- How does the patient walk?

Indoors

- Security;
- Obvious hazards;
- Warmth and type of heating. What access is there to switching the heating on?
- Evidence of uneaten food;
- Bad smells, e.g. body excreta or staining of clothes or floor from urine.

Health hazards

Safety hazards

The patient

- Greeting, mood, mental state;
- Colour;
- Warmth;
- Dress;
- State of wash, tidiness of person and whether well kempt;
- Cooking/shopping;
- Laundry;
- Furniture – height of chairs. The seat of the chair for an elderly

Name: Surname   Forename   M = Married
                                                  S = Single
                                                  W = Widowed

Address

GP

Date of birth

                                        Weight

Medical diagnoses/problems

1st Visit Health Visitor/Practice Nurse   Date

Accommodation: House/flat/bungalow/caravan/other

Facilities

Social contracts/isolation

Family support

Does impaired mental state affect independence?   Yes   No

Does poor motivation affect independence?   Yes   No

Does impairment of vision, speech, or hearing
affect independence?   Yes   No

Is patient independent for
Mobility indoors   Yes   No
Mobility outdoors   Yes   No
Dressing   Yes   No
Food   Yes   No
Toilet   Yes   No
Bathing   Yes   No
Household tasks   Yes   No
Finance   Yes   No
Aids   Yes   No
Treatments   Yes   No
2nd Visit Practice Nurse

Figure 7.4 Elderly survey: proforma.

person should be 18"–22" from the ground level. Height of bed
– should it be lowered?
– Self-alarm system.

Diagnosis and treatment of an illness is but one move forward
when assessing the overall needs of the elderly. The environment is
an important factor in planning the treatment and future management of the patient. The proforma given in Figure 7.4 provides a
useful means of summarizing the elderly patient's state of health
and physical surroundings or the completion of an action plan.

The examination

Physical check

– Test vision with card at three metres, with glasses. Specify if one
  or both eyes faulty;
– Check mouth and note dental caries, or inadequate dentures;
– Test hearing and use auriscope to check for wax;
– Check neck veins for rise of jugular venous pressure above
  clavicle;
– Check ankles for pitting oedema;
– Check vibration senses against tibial tuberosity and head of
  radius;
– Examine feet for corns, callouses and assess need for
  professional chiropody;
– Obtain specimen of urine and test, MSU should be taken later if
  indicated;
– Record blood pressure sitting;
– Check weight;
– Take blood for haemoglobin, ESR, urea and creatinine.

Symptomatic enquiry

1. Poor appetite;
2. Indigestion;
3. Loss of weight;
4. Productive cough;
5. Substernal pain;
6. Shortness of breath;

7. Painful joints;
8. Abnormal micturition;
9. Difficulty with bowels or diarrhoea;
10. Rectal or vaginal bleeding;
11. Other symptoms.

List of current medication and self-medication

Name of medicine or drug	Quantity and type	No. of Times daily

Doctor's check

— Cardiovascular system;
— Respiratory system;
— Gastro-intestinal;
— Central nervous system;
— Locomotor system;
— Smoking habits;
— Alcohol consumption.

Information and action

It is worth establishing your own local directory of services available for the elderly.

Keep your own at risk elderly register within the practice with easy access for all members of the Primary Health Care Team. Such a register should include all those patients who are in hospital or nursing homes.

Note that Age Concern has offices all over the country, and that British Telecom will fit amplifiers and press button telephones very readily.

WELL MAN CLINIC – MOT

Cardiovascular and coronary artery disease are the commonest cause of death in the western world. Predisposing factors are listed below.

Family history

A family history of coronary artery disease amongst first degree relatives puts young men at greater risk of developing this disease.

Hypertension

Hypertension predisoposes to an increased risk of death from cerebrovascular accident and coronary artery disease. It is now considered that raised systolic pressure as well as raised diastolic pressure are important predictors in coronary heart disease mortality.

Cigarette smoking

Smoking is one of the major causes of coronary heart disease. It accelerates the deposition of atheroma and reduces the oxygen carrying capacity of the red blood corpuscles. Smoking also interferes with normal lipid metabolism and causes vasoconstriction of the blood vessels.

Obesity

Associated with obesity are the risks of: hypertension; raised plasma cholesterol; and diabetes. These factors predispose to coronary heart disease.

Alcohol

Above average intake of alcohol results in: hypertension; obesity; and liver damage. These factors increase the risk of coronary heart disease.

Stress

It is very difficult to determine how significant stress is as a predisposing factor of coronary heart disease. A study monitoring stress is currently being undertaken by the Medical Research Council to try to determine the significance of this factor.

Diet

There is a strong correlation between the quantity of saturated fats eaten and mortality from coronary heart disease. Saturated fats eaten in above average amounts increase the total plasma level of cholesterol and also increases the low density lipoprotein, excess of which converts into atheroma. Figure 7.5 gives details of this process.

Aims of the MOT

- To identify those male patients within the practice who are at risk of coronary heart disease;
- To promote a low risk life-style;
- To initiate treatment for those patients at risk.

Health check

The following information will be recorded in the patients medical record. Practice protocols must be agreed before starting such a screening programme.

- Family history;
- General medical history;
- Smoking;
- Alcohol;
- Diet;
- Weight;
- Height;
- Exercise;
- Stress factors;
- Lung expansion;
- Urinalysis;
- Blood pressure;
- Blood lipid testing;
- Immunization status.

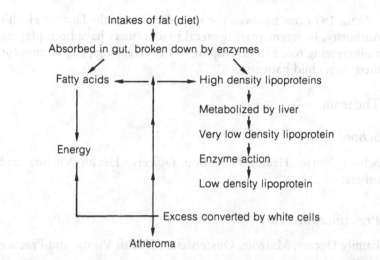

Intakes of fat (diet)

Absorbed in gut, broken down by enzymes

Fatty acids ← High density lipoproteins

Metabolized by liver

Very low density lipoprotein

Energy

Enzyme action

Low density lipoprotein

Excess converted by white cells

Atheroma

Figure 7.5 The process of fat metabolism. Cholesterol (a) membrane constituents; (b) synthesis of bile salts; (c) synthesis of adrenocorticoid hormone.

Recall

This should be done as agreed by the practice and detailed in the practice protocol.

Health education

It will be valuable to have a noticeboard displaying advice on giving-up smoking, on low cholesterol diets, and on reducing alcohol intake.

Having leaflets available within the practice as well as posters displaying areas of help may reinforce the importance of the screening.

The most effective method, however, is the face to face contact by health professionals – the doctor, the nurse and the health visitor.

CHILD DEVELOPMENT AND SURVEILLANCE

Prior to 1974 child health, including immunization, health education and surveillance, was the responsibility of the local authority.

Since 1974 this has been the responsibility of the District Health Authority. In recent years, general practitioners have been playing an increasing role and developing health screening programmes for their own child patients.

The team

School health

School Nurse, Health Education Officers, Health Visitors and others.

Pre-conceptual care

Family Doctor, Midwife, Obstetrician, Health Visitor and Practice Nurse.

Ante-natal care

Family Doctor, Midwife, Obstetrician, Health Visitor and Practice Nurse.

Intra-partum care

Midwife and/or Obstetrician.

Post-partum care

Midwife, Obstetrician and Health Visitor.

Child health and development

Health Visitor, General Practitioner or Clinical Medical Officers.

Call and recall

Many District Health Authorities are using a national child health computer system which consists of the following modules:

- A child register with neonatal data;
- Immunization;

- Pre-school health;
- School health.

Such computer records mean that:

- Health data cannot only be stored but also distributed to the family doctor and health visitor;
- Appointments for immunizations are sent directly to the health visitor who will arrange this with the child's parents or guardian, or an appointment is forwarded directly to the parent or guardian;
- Developmental health check appointments are arranged and an appointment sent directly;
- Lists of children due for specific screening tests are produced and teachers and school nurse are advised accordingly, e.g. Rubella.

Screening

The developmental screening examination and check provides a unique opportunity to determine not only the bonding relationship between mother and baby, but also provides the opportunity to detect any medical problems and helps in formulating relationships between patient and doctor and other members of the practice team.

Subsequent developmental screening provides the opportunity to assess the progress of a baby's increasing social and motor skills, as well as strengthening relations with the primary health care team. The schedule of screening recommended in the Court Report is given in Table 7.1.

The equipment needed at a child health clinic is listed below:

- Standard centile charts to plot weight and head circumference;
- Scales;
- Baby measuring [paedometer] tape, wall chart;
- Torch, ophthalmoscope;
- Stethoscope;
- Red brick/ball;
- Child's table and chairs to sit at;
- Stycar vision and hearing box.

The child's details should be regularly plotted on a Centile Dis-

Table 7.1 Schedule of screening recommended in the Court Report (1976). *Fit for the Future, Report on the committee on child health services,* HMSO, London

Age	Objectives and assessment
6–8 weeks	Assess mother and baby bonding
	Discuss feeding problems and check feeding
	Discuss immunization programme
	Exclude congenital abnormalities, such as dislocation of the hips
	Examine to make sure there is normal physical – neuro development
	Make sure the baby is registered with the practice
8–9 months	Carry out distraction hearing tests
	Determine the child can sit without support
	Assess manipulation skills
	Assess vision and test for squint
18 months	Ensure walking well
	Assess fine motor skills
2–3 years	Assess letter matching
	Vision testing (Snellen charts)
	Carry out word discrimination hearing test
	Assess speech and language
	Assess fine motor and performance skills

play Chart (Figure 7.6 for girls, Figure 7.7 for boys) which gives an indication of normal physical development.

Children with special needs

Under the Education Act 1981, those children who have special educational needs and whose needs cannot be met by the facilities of normal schools, have a statutory assessment and statement of needs made. This Act incorporates many of the recommendations of the Warnock Committee Report (1978) on the special educational needs of children.

As a result of the 1981 Act special education is available, although

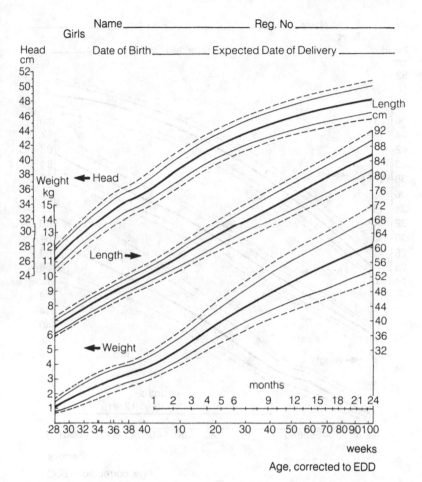

Figure 7.6 Centile display chart for girls.

not compulsory, for children from 2 years of age. The procedure for identifying special needs is as follows:

1. Assessment is carried out by a multi-disciplinary Child Development Team including Teacher, Educational Psychologist and a Doctor;
2. The medical report will include all specialist opinions and paramedical reports;
3. Parents can request this assessment whatever the age of the

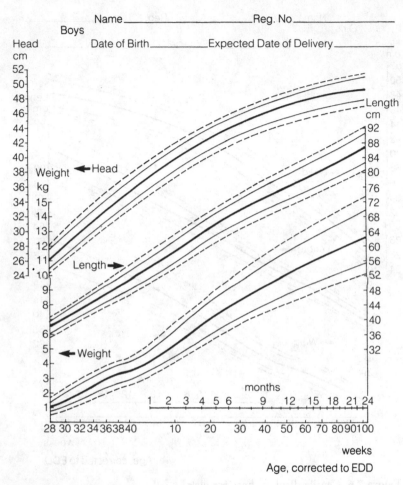

Figure 7.7 Centile display chart for boys.

child. The parent's consent is required if the child is under the age of 2 years;

4. A District Health Authority should inform the Educational Authority of any child it considers may be in need of special education;

5. The statement which is finally compiled is issued to parents and contains the parents' views of proposals for placement as well as the reports from the professionals.

The spirit of Warnock is that the handicapped child should be integrated into a normal school whenever possible. The child and the situation are then reviewed annually.

CHILD ABUSE

Child abuse, also known as non-accidental injury, is the deliberate injury of children usually by parents, caused by a variety of factors. Every year between three and five thousand children are known to be injured by their parents or guardians. The types of abuse are described below.

Physical abuse

Bruises

Minor bruises which show that the child may have been gripped tightly or shaken.

Facial bruises possibly caused by slapping or hitting the child. There may be 'finger bruising' in which the outlines of the fingers which slapped the child are clearly seen in the bruised area.

Bruising may occur over the bony prominences such as the ribs.

Lacerations

These may occur in any area, but in particular look for a torn upper lip frenum with swollen and bruised lips.

Scalds, burns, poisoning

Events which may happen particularly if the history is inadequate. Cigarette burns are important.

Bone and joint injuries

Ribs are frequently bruised or fractured and X-ray will show when injuries have occurred at different times. Fractured skull or long bones may also be present.

Human bites

Internal injuries

Drowning

Brain injuries

Emotional abuse

The child is continuously shouted at, criticized and blamed and often made a scapegoat.

Failure to thrive

Malnutrition

This may be suspected from slowness in reaching the development milestones.

Neglect

Lethargy, tiredness, withdrawn or very aggressive tendencies may all point to a history of neglect.

Sexual abuse

Sexual abuse is defined as the involvement of dependent, developmentally immature children and adolescents in sexual activities they do not truly comprehend, to which they are unable to give informed consent, or that violate the social taboos of family roles. Figure 7.8 shows the relationship of the abuser to the victim, and Figure 7.9 outlines the consequences of child sexual abuse.

Possible signs of sexual abuse are listed below:

- Regressive behaviours such as bed wetting;
- Sudden changes of mood;
- Excessive preoccupation with sexual matters;
- Sexually precocious;
- Hinting at the sex act by words, play actions or drawings;
- Change in eating habits, faddiness or loss of appetite;

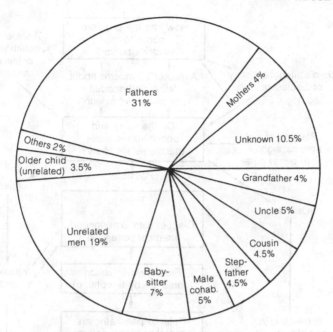

Figure 7.8 Child sexual abuse. The relationship of perpetrators to children of all ages. (Reproduced from: Hobbs, C.J. and Wynne, J.M. (1987) Child sexual abuse — an increasing rate of diagnosis. *The Lancet*, 10th October, 842–5.)

- Sleep disturbances, nightmares;
- Social withdrawal, isolation;
- Reluctance to participate in school activities or to change clothes for sports or gym;
- Avoidance of school medicals;
- Inappropriate displays of affection between father and daughter and mother and son;
- Truancy or deterioration in school performance;
- Recurrent urinary tract infections;
- Recurrent abdominal pain or headaches;
- Itching, soreness, discharge, bleeding, bruising and scratches of the anal/genital areas;
- Difficulty with walking and/or sitting;
- Disobedience, attention seeking, poor concentration;

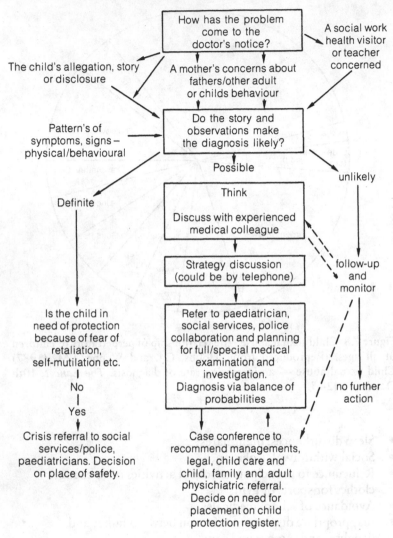

Figure 7.9 Flow chart showing possible outcomes of child sexual abuse. (From: Child Sexual Abuse, Initial Medical Contacts role. In *Diagnosis of Child Sexual Abuse: Guidance for Doctors*, HMSO, London.)

- Suicide attempt;
- Self-mutilation;
- Dependency on drugs, alcohol or solvents.

Pre-disposing factors to sexual abuse include:

Parents

- Very frequently have been abused themselves;
- Often the parents are very young. Many marry young;
- Many mothers are pregnant at the time;
- Parents have unrealistic expectations of their child;
- Invest everything in the marriage and child and then bills are unmet and housing circumstances may change and stress becomes the factor which causes the abuse;
- Overcrowding and unsatisfactory housing conditions;
- Unemployment;
- Poor health;
- Lack of affection or mothering in their own childhood;
- Lack trust;
- Those parents who abuse their child or children tend to attract similar partners;
- Inadequate emotionally.

Child

- Baby is wrong sex;
- Problems during pregnancy;
- Premature birth;
- Difficult labour or delivery;
- Unwanted pregnancy;
- Handicapped;
- Poor feeder;
- Lack of bonding;
- Irritable or 'colicky' baby;
- Child has behavioural problems;
- Illness.

Family

- Abusing families tend to have a variety of problems which seem to trap them;
- Poor relationships with other people;
- Difficulty in formulating any close relationship;
- These families are often isolated from their own family network and from their surrounding community;
- One problem seems to lead to another and the cycle tends to snowball.

Times in a day which can trigger event

Feeding

- Slow feeder;
- Baby frequently vomits;
- At weaning, and the toddler who refuses and spits the food out.

Crying

- Frequency of crying;
- Time of day;
- Persistent tone.

Napkin changing

Diagnosis and early recognition

The following injuries would arouse suspicion:

- Black eyes;
- Torn frenulum;
- Bruising of soft tissues;
- Bruising of back or chest;
- Burns or scalds, all of which do not match history;
- Fractures, especially in babies;
- Marks of the child or baby having been beaten with a stick or leather belt;
- Circular burns due to cigarettes;
- Bite marks;
- Sub-dural haematoma.

An abused child may appear as follows:

- Quiet;
- Small and thin for age;
- Withdrawn;
- Does not smile;
- Avoids eye contact;
- Wary of adults;
- 'Frozen watchfulness'.

In recognizing child abuse, the following aspects of its history should be taken into account:

- Age of child;
- Inconsistent story;
- Absence of explanation;
- History does not marry up with the findings on clinical examination;
- Delay in seeking treatment;
- Frequent attendance at the surgery for unrelated problems.

Emotional trauma

Emotional trauma may be suspected where there is:

1. Verbal aggression toward the child irrespective of behaviour;
2. The child is always wrong, ridiculed or mocked which results in the child being undermined and losing confidence;
3. Scapegoating – one child receives the blame until eventually he becomes the cause of all the problems;
4. A child who appears frightened, is soon in tears, lacks confidence, or is easily startled by noises. These children often stutter, appear shy and very often suck their thumb or bite their nails;
5. No eye to eye contact;
6. A child who avoids making relationships and prefers isolation whether it be with peers or adults;
7. A child who dislikes being touched;
8. Aggressive behaviour at times;
9. A child who is isolated at home and at school.

The cycle of deprivation

Abuse may lead the child into a cycle of deprivation which may manifest itself in physical and behavioural signs such as the following:

Physical

- Short stature;
- Pot belly;

- Hair dry, sparse, sometimes even bald patches;
- Small in bodily proportions;
- Hands, feet, legs and arms mottled and very cold;
- Hands and feet swollen because of vascular stasis;
- Small but multiple injuries apparent with bruising.

Behavioural

- Standing or sitting in one position for a long time;
- Rocking, head banging;
- Apathetic;
- Dejected;
- Frozen watchfulness – hypervigilance;
- Perverted appetite.

Action

In cases of actual or suspected non-accidental injury to children or child abuse, the following action needs to be taken by agencies and members of the public.

Safety of the child is of paramount concern. The timing of an application for a Place of Safety Order, if necessary, is a matter for the officer of the authorized agency concerned.

A member of the public may suspect abuse or injury to a child and contact any of the agencies. The identity of this person must remain anonymous initially, if requested. The informant may be asked to make a statement and give evidence if Court proceedings follow. The authorized agencies are: Department of Social Services; Police; and NSPCC. Non-authorized agencies are: General Practitioner; Health Visitor; Teacher; Probation Service.

Authorized agencies must investigate immediately by contacting and informing other two authorized agencies in order to:

- Check whether already known;
- Inform about action being taken;
- Ensure safety by a Place of Safety Order or Care Proceedings brought into effect by Department of Social Services; or the Police; or the NSPCC.

A Place of Safety Order may precede the medical investigations, in which case these should be carried out immediately the child is received at the Place of Safety. If there is obvious injury the child will be referred to hospital.

The next step is for the Senior Social Worker to call a Case Conference. All the agencies involved will decide at the case conference whether the child's name is *not* to be placed on the NAIC register; or the child's name *is* to be placed on the NAIC register, and the category:

- Non-accidental injury;
- Suspected non-accidental injury;
- Physical neglect;
- Failure to thrive;
- Emotional abuse;
- Sexual abuse;
- High degree of risk;
- Where the child is in an environment where previous abuse has occurred.

At the case conference the supervising agency and keyworker will be decided upon and further appropriate action wil be agreed, with both short-term and long-term objectives being set.

The supervising agency then sends details for insertion into the NAIC Register which is held by the Department of Social Services, and makes sure the family doctor is informed. The supervising agency subsequently maintains contact with the case and the child's care.

When the risk is assumed to be over the child's name is removed from the Register, a decision which is only taken after a case conference to which all agencies previously involved are invited to attend together with those who may have become involved.

FURTHER READING

Well Man Clinic – MOT

Coronary Heart Disease – The Need for Action (1987) A Report from the Office of Health Economics. The OHE London, England.
Community Prevention and Control of Cardiovascular Diseases (1988) Technical Report Series 732, WHO, Geneva.
Coronary Heart Disease – Reducing the Risk (1987) Open University, John Wiley & Sons Ltd.

Kannel, W.B., *et al.* (1973) Cholesterol in the production of atherosclerotic disease. New perspectives based in the Framingham Study. *Annals of Internal Medicine*, **90**, 85.

Holbrook, J.H., Grundy S.M., Hennekens, C.H. *et al.* Cigarette smoking and cardiovascular diseases. A statement from the health professionals by a task force appointed by the steering committee of the American Heart Association. *Circulation*, **70**, 1114A–1117A.

Diet and Cardiovascular Disease (1985) DHSS, HMSO, London.

Heart Attacks: Prevention and Treatment (1979) BMA.

Available from:
Family Doctor Publications,
BMA House,
Tavistock Square,
London, WC1H 9JP.

Promoting Better Health (1987) The Government's Programme for Improving Health Care, HMSO, London.

Randle, P.S. (1985) *The Coma Report: Diet and Cardiovascular Disease.* DHSS, HMSO, London.

Fullard, E., Fowler, G. and Gray, M. (1987) Promoting prevention in primary care: controlled trial of low-technology low-cost approach, *British Medical Journal*, **294**, 1080–2.

Rent-an-audit: an educational exercise facilitating change (1987) *European Newsletter on Quality Assurance*, **4**, 5.

Useful address

The Oxford Centre for Prevention in Primary Care,
Radcliffe Infirmary,
Woodstock Road,
Oxford, OX2 6HE.
Telephone: 0865 24891 Ext. 4427

Child development and surveillance

Sheridan, M.D. (1975) *From Birth to Five Years: Children's Developmental Progress*, 3rd Edn, Nfer-Nelson, Windsor.

Holt, K.S. (1977) *Developmental Paediatrics* Butterworth, London.

The Standing Medical Advisory Committee and The Standing Nursing and Midwifery Advisory Committee (1986) *Screening for the Detection of Congential Dislocation of the Hip*, DHSS, London.

The General Medical Services Committee of the British Medical Association and The Royal College of General Practitioners (1984) *Handbook of Preventive Care for Pre-school Children*, London.

Illingworth, R.S. (1983) *The Development of the Infant and Young Child*, 8th Edn, Churchill Livingstone, London.

Polnay, L. and Hull D. (1985) *Community Paediatrics*, Churchill Livingstone, London.

Useful address

Screening equipment can be obtained from:
National Foundation for Educational Research,
The Mere,
Upton Park,
Slough,
Bucks.
Telephone: WINDSOR: 858961
STYCAR VISION BOX
        HEARING BOX

Child abuse

Finkelhor, D. and Associates (1986) *A Sourcebook on Child Sexual Abuse*, Sage Publications, London.

Mrazek, P.B., Lynch, M. and Bentovim, A. (1981) A recognition of child sexual abuse in the United Kingdom. In: (eds P.B. Mrazek and C.H. Kempe) *Sexually Abused Children and their Families*, Pergamon Press, London.

Mrazek, D. and Mrazek, P.B. (1985) Child maltreatment. In: (eds M. Rutter and L. Herson) *Child and Adolescent Psychiatry: Modern Approaches*, Blackwell, Oxford.

Kempe, R.S. and Kempe, C.H. (1984) *Sexual Abuse of Children and Adolescents*, Freeman, New York.

Schechter, M.D. and Roberge, L. (1976) Sexual exploitation. In: (eds R.E. Helfer and C.H. Kempe) *Child Abuse and Neglect: the Family and the Community*, Ballinger, Cambridge, Mass.

DHSS (1988) *Diagnosis of Child Sexual Abuse: Guidance for Doctors*, HMSO, London.

Markove, H. (1988) The frequency of child sexual abuse in the UK. *Healthy Trends No. 1*, 20, 2–6.

Child Abuse – Working Together. DHSS guidelines.
HC [88] 38/LAC [88] 10.

Training Resources

Sexually Abused Children – The Sensitive Medical Examination and Management. VHS video and booklet available from:
Royal Society of Medicine,
RSM Services Limited,
Film and Television Unit,
1, Wimpole Street,
London, W1M 8AE.
Telephone: 01-499 7422

VHS videos and accompanying booklets on child abuse available from:
Audio Visual Service
University of Leeds
Leeds LS2 9JT
Telephone: 0532 431751

A database of information on training materials, courses and literature is available on request at:
The Development Officer,
National Children's Bureau,
8, Wakley Street,
London, EC1V 7QE.

Distance learning pack on child abuse available through:
The Open University,
Walton Hall,
Milton Keynes,
MK7 6KK.

Useful addresses

1. Your own Dept. of Social Services
2. NSPCC branch

National Society for Prevention of Cruelty to Children,
National Headquarters,
67, Saffron Hill,
London, EC1.

London Communication Centre,
Enquiries, information and advice,
24 hr service: 01-404 4447.

8

Promotion of health and prevention of disease

HEALTH EDUCATION AND HEALTH PROMOTION

The Government's recent White Paper *Promoting Better Health*, 1987 and the DHSS Circular *Community Nursing Services and Primary Health Care Teams*, 1987 both placed emphasis on the need to promote health and prevent illness. This dual approach to health care has been followed since 1968 by the Health Education Authority which has been working for better health in the United Kingdom.

Financed by the Government, the Health Education Authority educates, campaigns, sponsors research and publishes authoritative advice on a wide range of issues concerned with health.

The Authority itself is an independent body of distinguished men and women from different professional backgrounds appointed by the Secretary of State for Social Services.

The Health Education Authority's activities are divided into programmes which cover either areas of health or groups of people.

Health education

Health education aims to provide information to ensure that all members of the public can with competence: act upon the knowledge provided; use all the facilities of the health care system; and understand those factors which can affect health such as smoking, alcohol abuse, nutrition, and stress.

Health promotion

Health promotion is much more involved in helping the individual to take responsibility for their own health and to make positive changes for a healthier life style.

The *Ottowa Charter for Health Promotion* was compiled and agreed at the World Health Organization's Conference in Canada in 1986. This defined health promotion as '... the process of enabling people to increase control over and improve their health.'

Campaign areas

The Health Education Authority's activities are detailed below in terms of the main areas of health or groups of people at which its campaigns are aimed.

Smoking

This is the biggest preventable cause of death and disease in Britain. Campaigns are mounted to persuade smokers to give up and youngsters not to start. Research is sponsored to determine the most effective way to get people to give up smoking; and National No Smoking Day is promoted each March.

Heart disease

Since smoking increases the risk of heart disease, programmes to tackle these two areas often run concurrently. Education is provided on risks and also on preventative measures such as exercise; healthy diet; regular screening; and removing stress.

Alcohol, drugs and other addictions

The Health Education Authority's message on alcohol is advice on safe limits which allows enjoyment without harm. It is also co-operating with the Government in the national fight against hard drugs and solvent abuse.

Dental health

Education for dental health is aimed principally at young people and mothers with newborn babies, so that good health and dental care can be set early in life. In addition, dentists are being encouraged to be more educational in their approach to their patients.

Family and personal health

The key campaign areas in this broad category are:

- Health in pregnancy;
- Health of pre-school children;
- Asian Mother and Baby Campaign – with publications and learning packages in different languages;
- Sexual health – covering contraception and prevention of infection;
- Family planning – the Health Education Authority, along with the Family Planning Association provides a family planning information service. This offers a countrywide information service, a resource and information centre and a range of publications;
- AIDS and homosexuality.

Health education for young people

The Health Education Authority views school health as crucial.

Adult and community education

The Health Education Authority, along with the Open University has developed educational programmes designed to help people to lead a healthy life and make them aware of issues which affect health.

Health and old age

'Age Well' is the slogan under which the Health Education Authority sets out to encourage a positive approach to health among the elderly. As well as advising individuals, the Authority is encouraging

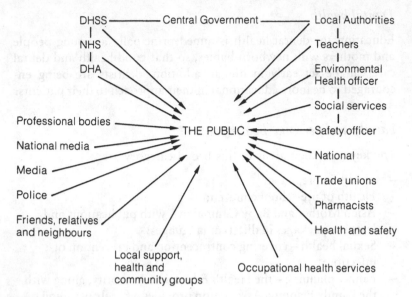

Figure 8.1 The interrelationship between professional and educational groups involved in health education for the public.

self-help group projects, and offering help to those who care for our senior citizens.

Professional development

If the public are the main focus of the Authority's advice, the support and development of professional workers in a position to influence the public is equally crucial. The Health Education Authority works closely with many professional and educational groups. The interrelationships are illustrated in Figure 8.1.

The Health Education Officer

There are some 500 Health Education Officers in post in the United Kingdom at the present time. The role of the Health Education Officer is summarized in Figure 8.2. They work from health education/promotion centres within the health authority, but not all Health Authorities have such centres.

These centres are the focal point for health promotion in an area,

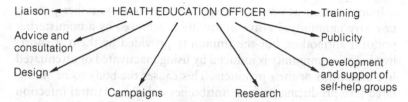

Figure 8.2 The role of the health education office.

and provide a variety of teaching aids and publicity material promoting aspects of health. Some centres are also responsible for training and run multidisciplinary as well as specific discipline courses. They are also the focal point for community liaison, often promoting health through a community newsletter.

In conclusion, it can be said that common to all the activities and programmes of the Health Education Authority and its Officers is the belief that increased understanding can lead to change, both in the way people behave and in the social factors which can contribute to ill health.

IMMUNIZATION AGAINST INFECTIOUS DISEASES – CHILDREN

This section covers immunization from birth to leaving school. Within the practice a doctor may delegate responsibility for immunization to a nurse provided the following conditions are fulfilled:

1. The nurse is willing to be professionally accountable for this work within the practice;
2. The nurse has received training and is competent in all aspects of immunization, including contraindications;
3. Training has been given in the recognition and treatment of anaphylaxis;
4. There is an agreed practice protocol on such issues as:
    (a) What the agreed policy is if a child or baby attends with other than a parent;
    (b) Agreement on site(s) of injection for immunization following the Department of Health's guidelines;
    (c) Whether written consent should be obtained from the parent before giving an injection;
    (d) With whom the practice nurse should check the vaccine.

Immunization against infectious diseases conveys either passive or active immunity. Passive immunity is achieved by administering preform antibodies, but the immunity provided by them is short-lived. Active immunity is induced by using inactivated or attenuated live organisms or their products. This causes the body to be stimulated into producing its own antibodies either by natural infection or by vaccine. The immunity so gained can be longlasting and enhanced by further exposure to the organism.

Type of vaccine preparation

Vaccines are either viral or bacterial in origin and are grouped according to whether they are:

1. Live;
2. Inactivated;
3. Toxoid.

Group	Viral vaccines	Bacterial vaccines
Live	Rubella	BCG
	Mumps	
	Measles, mumps, rubella	
	Oral polio	
Inactivated		Pertussis
Toxoid		Diptheria
		Tetanus

Live vaccines

Live vaccines are prepared from attenuated strains of organisms usually freeze-dried so that they will remain viable for long periods provided they are kept at low temperatures.

Clinical effects produced by live vaccines may resemble those of the natural disease but are usually much milder. A simple administration of the live vaccine usually produces long-term immunity.

Oral polio contains vaccines prepared from virus serotypes and for this reason it has to be given more than once to ensure an adequate response to each virus serotype.

Inactivated vaccines

Inactivated vaccines consist of killed organisms from bacteria. There is no replication of the organism within the body, and any reactions produced do not simulate those observed during the natural course of the natural disease.

Inactivated vaccines are administered more than once to ensure an adequate antibody response.

Different vaccines require different intervals between doses. Delaying administration of the second dose for at least six weeks and the third for 6–12 months enhances the antibody response and results in viable immunity.

Schedule of immunization

Immunization should be given to protect those age groups most susceptible to the natural infection. The schedule recommended by the DHSS is as follows:

First year of life

13 weeks (3 months)	Diptheria, tetanus, pertussis and polio
19–21 weeks (4–5 months) That is, 6–8 weeks later	Diptheria, tetanus, pertussis and polio
36–40 weeks (8–11 months) That is, 4–6 months later	Diptheria, tetanus, pertussis and polio

Notes

If pertussis is contraindicated or declined, diptheria and tetanus may be given alone. In a pertussis epidemic, intervals may be 4 weeks with a further dose of diptheria and tetanus 12–18 months later.

1–5 years

To be given at 12–15 months, or 4–5 years if not previously given.	Measles/mumps/rubella (MMR)

Notes

Ignore history of measles or measles immunization alone.

School entry

4–5 years	Diptheria, tetanus and oral polio booster

Notes

Pertussis may be given up to the 6th birthday if this has been declined earlier.

Measles/mumps/rubella and diptheria and tetanus may be given either at the same time in different sites or one month apart.

10–15 years

Girls only	Rubella

Notes

Ignore history of rubella infection. The current recommendation is that the rubella vaccine to be given at this age, even if child had MMR in infancy.

11–13 years

All	BCG Leave 6 weeks after varicella, rubella, measles or their vaccines, as response is reduced.

Notes

For tuberculin negative or Grade 1 only, unless given at birth in families at risk.

No immunization in that arm for 3 months.

School leavers

All	Tetanus and polio boosts. Tetanus not within 5 years of previous boost.

Contraindications

Immunization is contraindicated in general by acute febrile illness. The following specific contraindications relate to the immunization being given.

Pertussis

- Cerebral irritation or damage in the neonate;
- Severe reaction to previous dose (local or general reaction);
- History of fits or neurological disease;
- Idiopathic epilepsy in parents or siblings.

Tetanus

- Not within five years of previous dose;
- Febrile illness;
- Serious general or local reaction to a previous dose;

'Flu

- Not under four years of age or as recommended annually by Department of Health letter;
- Hypersensitivity to egg, polymyxin or neomycin.

Polio

- Immunological deficiency;
- Gastro-intestinal symptoms;
- Severe hypersensitivity to polymyxin, neomycin, penicillin or streptomycin;
- Malignant conditions such as lymphoma, leukaemia,
- Hodgkin's disease and other tumours of the reticulo-endothelial system.

Diptheria

- A live vaccine within three weeks of another live vaccine, unless simultaneously given in another limb;
- Malignancy or tumours of reticulo-endothelial system;
- Hypogammaglobulinaemia;
- Corticosteroid treatment;
- Immunosuppressive treatment;
- Radiation.

Rubella

- Within six weeks of immunoglobulin or blood plasma;
- Sensitivity to neomycin or polymyxin;
- Allergy;
- Thrombocytopenia;
- Had an infection within the last three weeks;
- Patients who are receiving high doses of corticosteroid or immunosuppressive treatment including radiation;
- Patients suffering from Hodgkin's disease or other tumours of the reticulo-endothelial system.

Measles/mumps/rubella

- Severe acute respiratory infection;
- Untreated malignant disease;
- Patients with impaired immunity or on immunosuppressive therapy;
- Live vaccine injection during the previous three weeks;
- Hypersensitivity to neomycin, kanamycin and egg products or patients with a history of anaphylaxis.

Administration

The following questions should be asked before administering any immunizations

- Is the baby ill or unwell in any way?
- Has the baby had side-effects from any previous immunization?
- Has the baby or anyone in the immediate family ever had fits or convulsions?

- Is the baby developing normally?
- Were there any problems with the baby during the first week of life?

Before giving the immunization, the following points should be checked.

1. The leaflets supplied with the vaccine should be read;
2. The identity of the vaccine must be checked to ensure the right product is used for each occasion;
3. The expiry date must be noted and checked;
4. The batch number must be recorded in the patient's notes;
5. The recommended storage conditions must be adhered to.

Dose

Oral polio vaccine (live)

Oral administration
3 drops dose

Inactivated polio vaccine

Deep subcutaneous or intramuscular injection
0.5 ml dose
23G needle size

Diptheria/tetanus/pertussis or diptheria/tetanus

Deep subcutaneous or intramuscular injection
0.5 ml dose
23G needle size

Measles/mumps/rubella

Deep subcutaneous or intramuscular injection
0.5 ml dose
23G needle size

Reconstitution of vaccines

- The diluent supplied with the freeze-dried vaccine should only be used when reconstituting the vaccine;
- The colour of the product must be checked to make sure it is as stated by the manufacturers in the accompanying leaflet;
- A 21G needle and 1 ml syringe should be used to reconstitute the vaccine;
- A 23G or needle should be used to administer the product.

Cleaning of skin

The skin should be cleaned with, for example, mediswabs, but the alcohol must be allowed to evaporate before injection of the vaccine since alcohol at the site of the injection can inactivate live vaccine preparations.

Route of administration

Oral polio vaccine must only be given by mouth.

If a sugar lump is used to administer the polio vaccine, the sugar lump should be prepared immediately before administration. Allowing pre-prepared sugar lumps to stand at room temperature for some time may reduce the efficacy of the vaccine.

Intramuscular or deep subcutaneous injection should be used for all vaccines. In infants, the antero-lateral aspect of the thigh or upper arm are the sites of choice. If the buttock is used where there is any amount of fatty tissue it is considered that the efficacy of the vaccine may be reduced.

Records

Thorough records should be kept of immunizations, as follows:

- A record should be kept in the patient's record of each dose of vaccine administered giving the date, type of vaccine, batch no., dose given and route;

- Information should also be entered in the District Health Authority Child Health Record (these records are forwarded to the school the child first attends);
- Enter on, parents record of child's immunization;
- Enter on age-sex register;
- Inform District Health Authority computer;
- Enter on practice computer;
- Complete appropriate form for Family Practitioner Committee in the form of FP73 or 73(a) or 73(b).

Communication through the practice

The public can be informed of the immunization programme which is available through a variety of ways:

- Ante-natal groups;
- Post-natal groups;
- Opportunistically at clinics such as well woman, pre-conceptual and family planning;
- Posters and leaflets displayed focusing on one illness, such as measles/mumps/rubella;
- Using the practice noticeboard;
- Practice newsletter;
- Practice booklet or leaflet.

The following audio-visual aids are all related to preventative care in the form of an immunization programme, and are obtainable from a local Health Education Office.

Leaflets

- Immunization;
- Measles/mumps/rubella;
- Rubella for parents and their daughters;
- Pertussis.

Posters

- All subjects.

Videos

- Rubella;
- Advice to parents;
- Pertussis.

Leaflets for the child and the parents relating to rubella with a rubella carrying card are available from:

Leaflets Unit,
DHSS,
Government Buildings,
Honeypot Lane,
Stanmore,
Middlesex,
HA7 122.

HEPATITIS

Hepatitis is an infection of the liver caused by a virus. There are three main types of the disease: hepatitis A, hepatitis B, and non A and non B hepatitis.

Hepatitis A

Yellow jaundice was recognized first by Hippocrates. The specific virus causing 'infectious hepatitis' was first recognized in 1973. It is usually transmitted via the faecal-oral route and is more common in conditions of over-crowding and poor sanitation. Hepatitis A has an incubation period of four weeks.

All age groups are susceptible but the highest incidence is known to be in school-age children and young adults. In tropical countries the peak of reported infection occurs during the rainy season.

Prevention and control of hepatitis A is difficult. Spread of the virus can be reduced by carrying out hygienic measures and the proper disposal of excreta.

The giving of human immunoglobulin affords short-term protection for those travellers going to countries where the condition is endemic.

Patients who are unfortunate enough to contract hepatitis A may be unwell and incapacitated for many weeks. The condition does not usually lead to chronic or permanent liver damage. Morbidity is relatively low.

Hepatitis B

Hepatitis B was first recognized at the turn of the century. It was not until 1967–8 that a specific marker for hepatitis B, Australian Antigen, was identified. Figure 8.3 shows the structure of the hepatitis B virus, and Table 8.1 explains the terminology used in this disease.

The incidence is high in tropical and developing countries and in some areas of Europe. In the British Isles, transmisson of the virus is through blood or blood products.

Those persons infected early in life may become persistent carriers. The range of possible consequences from HBV infection is given in figure 8.4.

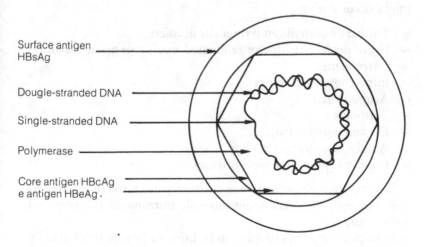

Surface antigen
HBsAg

Dougle-stranded DNA

Single-stranded DNA

Polymerase

Core antigen HBcAg
e antigen HBeAg .

Figure 8.3 The structure of HBV.

Table 8.1 *Terminology used in connection with hepatitis B*

Abbreviation	Meaning
HBV	Hepatitis B virus (or the Dane Particle)
HBsAg	Hepatitis B surface antigen (or Australian Antigen)
HBcAg	Hepatitis B core antigen
HBeAg	The 'e' antigen associated with the core
Anti-HBs	Antibody-to-hepatitis B surface antigen
Anti-HBc	Antibody-to-hepatitis B core antigen
Anti-HBe	Antibody to the 'e' antigen

The incubation period is probably six weeks to six months and it occurs in specific high risk groups.

Hepatitis B has a high mortality rate.

Modes of transmission of hepatitis B

Hepatitis B can be transmitted directly through the skin by inoculation of contaminated blood, however minute. This inoculation might occur during:

- The use of unsterilized syringes or needles;
- Use of inadequately decontaminated surgical or gynaecological instruments;
- Intravenous drug abuse;
- Acupuncture;
- Tattooing;
- Ear and nose piercing;
- Accidents with razor blades;
- Contamination from toothbrushes.

In some countries where these customs persist, the ritual circumcision of male or female using unsterile instruments is a potential risk factor.

In tropical countries people can be infected by repeated biting by bloodsucking insects.

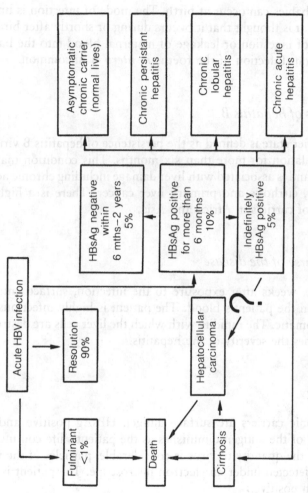

Figure 8.4 Possible consequences of HBV infection.

Transmission can also occur during transfer of body secretions; by biting an infected person; and through intimate contact.

Perinatal transmission of hepatitis B virus from carrier mothers to their babies can occur at birth. The mode of infection is uncertain, but it is thought that it occurs during or shortly after birth as a result of ingestion or leakage of maternal blood into the baby's circulation. Infection of the foetus *in utero* is uncommon.

Carriers of hepatitis B

The carrier state is defined as the persistence of hepatitis B virus in the circulation for more than six months. This condition may be lifelong and is associated with liver damage including chronic active hepatitis, cirrhosis and primary liver cancer. There is a high incidence of carriers in Africa and Asia.

The course of the disease

From six weeks after exposure to the infection, surface antigens appear in the patient's blood. The patient is highly infectious but asymptomatic. The rapidity with which the liver cells are destroyed determines the severity of the hepatitis.

Serology

All chronic carriers are surface antigen HBsAg positive and the quantity of the antigen diminishes as the patient's life continues.

When the quantity of virus is considerable, particles of the virus can be detected under an electron microscope. The patient is also e antigen positive.

Prevention

All members of the public who kindly donate blood have their blood tested for the hepatitis B surface antigen.

Correct labelling of infected material, according to those agreed protocols within the health district, should prevent accidental infection.

Passive immunization

High titre hepatitis B immunoglobulin which has been prepared from selected plasma containing the hepatitis B surface antibody can be given to confer temporary passive immunity under certain conditions.

1. Indications
    (a) Single acute exposure to hepatitis B virus, such as occurs when
         (i)   blood containing the surface antigen is inoculated
         (ii) blood containing the surface antigen is ingested
         (iii) blood containing the surface antigen is splashed onto the conjunctiva;
    (b) Prophylactic dose of hepatitis B immunoglobulin should be given to babies at risk of infection with hepatitis B virus. The dose of hepatitis B immunoglobulin should be given as soon as possible after birth of within 12 hours of birth. If this practice is adhered to it is estimated that the risk of the baby becoming a carrier is reduced by approximately 70%. More recently it has been recommended that the combination of passive and active immunization be adopted. By using both it has been estimated that the risk of being a carrier is reduced by 90%. The dose of hepatitis B immunoglobulin that is recommended for the newborn is 1–2 ml (200 iu of anti-hepatitis B per ml).
2. Dose for adults
    The optimal dose has not been established. The range is 250–500 iu. The hepatitis B immunoglobulin should be administered as soon after exposure as possible and preferably within 48 hours. The first dose should not be administered more than 7 days after exposure. It is generally recommended that two doses of hepatitis B immunoglobulin should be given 30 days apart.

Active immunization

HB Vax and Engerix B vaccines should be stored between 2–8°C but not frozen. They each contain 20 micrograms of hepatitis virus per millilitre and should only be given intramuscularly.

Prior to commencing a vaccination programme, the patient should have a blood test (10 ml) to determine whether the patient is already surface antibody positive. If the patient is surface antibody positive, no vaccination is required. If not, a course of three vaccinations should be commenced.

The vaccine should be well shaken and injected into the deltoid muscle of an adult or the antero-lateral aspect of the thigh of infants or children.

The dose for adults in 1 ml and for children 0.5 ml. The interval between the first dose and the second dose should be one month, and the third dose should be given six months after the first dose. Two months after the third dose, blood should be tested to ascertain whether the vaccine has sero-converted. If a good response is not obtained a booster dose should be given, and a further blood test taken two months after the booster dose. A good response is 100 iu/ml.

Non-responders must be protected by passive immunization if inoculation occurs. It is estimated that some 15% of individuals do not respond after three injections. Most of these are over 40 years of age and a higher proportion are women.

The duration of immunity is not known and it is advisable to retest after five years and give a booster dose of vaccine if antibody levels have dropped below 50 iu/ml.

Side-effects of the vaccine are very rare but a localized redness and soreness at the site of the injection may occur.

The pregnant woman or nursing mother or any patient with an acute infection should not be vaccinated.

Personnel at risk

The following lists show the categories of people at risk of contracting hepatitis B.

(a) *Health care personnel* – especially those in contact with blood and needles.

- Surgeons and members of the surgical team;
- Anaesthetists;
- Gastroenterologists;
- Intensive care teams;
- Laboratory workers;
- Accident and emergency staff;
- Midwives and nurses;
- Renal unit staff;
- Medical students;
- Nurses and staff working with the mentally handicapped and mentally ill people because of the risk of introducing infection from bites.

(b) *Community health care personnel*

- General Practitioners;
- Practice Nurses;
- District Nurses;
- Midwives;
- Community Psychiatric Nurses.

(c) *Others*

- Staff working in prisons;
- Staff working in homes for the mentally handicapped;
- Workmen, cleaners and laundry workers in above situations;
- Staff treating patients with haemophilia and other centres providing regular treatment with blood or blood products;
- Dentists and ancillary staff;
- Ambulancemen;
- Long-term prisoners;
- Policemen;
- Blood transfusion staff;
- Drug addicts;
- Sexually promiscuous individuals – male homosexuals, prostitutes;
- Patients undergoing haemodialysis or transplant surgery;
- Travellers to high endemic areas, especially Africa and India where infection is additionally considered to be transmitted via mosquitoes and bed bugs;

- Patients requiring frequent blood transfusions;
- Infants born to carrier mothers;
- Chiropodists;
- Tattooists;
- Mortuary workers and embalmers;
- Military personnel who serve in high risk areas;
- Patients with natural or acquired immune deficiency;
- Staff at sexually transmitted disease centres/special clinics;
- Patients suffering from Down's Syndrome because these patients have a defective immune response and are easily infected and become carriers.

Non A non B hepatitis

This type of hepatitis has relatively recently been diagnosed. Diagnosis is made when the patient has the signs of hepatitis but virus A and virus B of hepatitis cannot be isolated.

FURTHER READING

Health Education and health promotion

Promoting Better Health (1987) The Government's Programme for Improving Primary Health Care. HMSO, London.
DHSS Health Services Development. *Community Nursing Services and Primary Health Care Teams* (1987) HC(87)29:HC(FP)(98)10. DHSS, London.
Journal of the Institute of Health Education
Health Education News

Other sources of information

Learning Materials for Community, Adult and Health Education,
Learning Materials Service Office,
The Open University,
PO Box 188,
Milton Keynes,
MK7 6DH.

The Open University
Department of Health and Social Welfare
Newspaper

Education for Health through the *Primary Health Care Project* (developed
by the Open University in conjunction with the Health Education
Council)

- Abuse in Families;
- A Systematic Approach to Nursing Care;
- Mental Handicap: Patterns for Living;
- Rehabilitation;
- Coronary Heart Disease;
- Caring for Older People;
- Caring for Children and Young People;
- Mental Health and Mental Illness;
- Drug Use and Misuse.

Guidelines for the safe decontamination of instruments and appliances can
be obtained from:

The Department of Health,
14 Russell Square,
London, WC1B 5EP.

A report *An Evaluation of Portable Steam Sterilisers for Unwrapped Instruments and Utensils* is published as Health Equipment Information
No. 185, (July 1988).
Letter from the Department of Health on the decontamintion of instruments and appliances used in the vagina (December, 1988) gives details
of recommended methods to be used.

Immunization against infectious diseases – children

Department of Health (1988) *Immunization against infectious disease*,
HMSO, London.

Hepatitis

Hepatitis Nursing in the UK (1987) Report of the Wembley Conference,
Royal College of Nursing.

Viral Hepatitis in Britain (1975) Office of Health Economics, Report.
Immunization against Infectious Diseases (1988) Department of Health
and Social Security, HMSO, London.

9

Clinics for special groups of people

This chapter describes the requirements for setting up and running various clinics for special groups of people within a practice. The topics covered are:

- Well woman;
- Smoking;
- Diabetes;
- Pre-conceptual care;
- Alcohol;
- Foreign travel;
- AIDS.

WELL WOMAN SCREENING

Well woman clinics not only provide a screening programme, but also afford a unique opportunity for patients to share worries which are immediate or longstanding. The Practice Nurse, by organizing a well woman clinic, can help the female patient in a variety of ways by identifying problems, giving informed advice and referring as necessary. The aims of such a clinic are:

- To provide a needed service to women that is acceptable to all women;
- To provide screening;
- To provide participatory health education with patient-centred outcomes;
- To provide an environment conducive to changing health behaviour;
- To provide follow-up and referral as appropriate;

- To support self-help groups;
- To involve the primary care team members in support groups.

The following topics should be included in a well woman clinic:

1. *Clinical procedures*
   - Weight;
   - Height;
   - Urinalysis;
   - Blood pressure;
   - Breast screening;
   - Cervical smear screening.
2. *General health and wellbeing*
   - Diet – related to findings from weight and height;
   - Contraception and family planning help;
   - Psychosexual problems;
   - Menopausal problems or worries;
   - Menstrual worries;
   - Relationships and marital problems;
   - Ante-natal care and parentcraft classes;
   - Post-natal care and support groups;
   - Rubella immunization – patient advised to avoid pregnancy for 3 months after immunization.

The rest of this section will focus on breast screening and cervical smear screening.

Breast screening

Statistics show that while some 2000 women a year die in the UK from carcinoma of the cervix, nearly 15 000 – eight times that number – die from carcinoma of the breast. It is of interest to note that a majority of the women who attend regularly for a cervical smear test admit to never examining their own breasts.

The Government has made monies available for health authorities to set up a national breast screening programme for women aged 50–65 years. These patients will be invited to attend for breast screening through Family Practitioner Committees, similar to the system which Family Practitioner Committees operate for calling and recalling women for cervical smear screening.

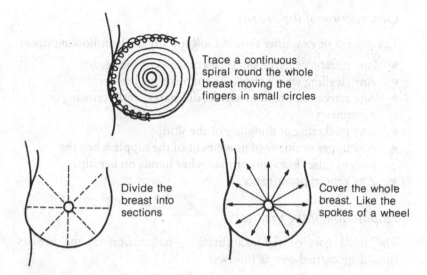

Trace a continuous spiral round the whole breast moving the fingers in small circles

Divide the breast into sections

Cover the whole breast. Like the spokes of a wheel

Figure 9.1 Methods of examining the breast.

Examination of the breasts

The patient should be taught *self-examination* of her breasts (Figure 9.1). She should be instructed to examine her breasts regularly, either (1) immediately post menses, or (2) on the same date each month if post-menopausal.

The patient should be taught that examination of the breasts includes three aspects, all of which are equally important, namely: (1) Inspection; (2) Observation; (3) Palpitation.

Inspection of the breasts

The method for inspection of the breasts is as follows:

First, instruct the patient to sit upright, unclothed to the waist and examine her breasts and their contours: demonstrate how she can do this at home in front of a mirror.

Secondly, instruct the patient to lift both arms straight above the head palms facing forward. This stretches the pectoralis major muscles and causes the breasts to become more prominent. If the patient is unable to raise both arms above the head, she can place her hands on her hips and press inwards with the elbows back. Alternatively, the patient can place her hands on her head.

Observation of the breasts

The patient or examiner should look for any of the following signs:

- Any difference in the shape or contours of the breast;
- Any swelling which alters the shape of the breasts;
- Any retraction of either nipple, discharge, rash, crusting or asymmetry;
- Any puckering or dimpling of the skin;
- Any upper or outward movement of the nipple when the patient raises her arms or places her hands on her hips;
- Any venous prominence.

Palpatation of the breasts

The third part of the examination, palpitation of the breasts should be carried out as follows:

Ask the patient to lie down on the couch with a pillow supporting the head; she may need a folded towel or small pillow under the shoulder on the side of examination. This helps to spread the breast tissue out and aids examination.

Ask the patient to roll slightly over to one side so that the nipple of the first breast to be examined is approximately in the centre. The larger and more pendulous the breasts the more the patient will need to roll over.

Palpate all parts of the breast using the soft fleshy flat part of the fingers. The breast may divided into quadrants or the breast may be examined tracing a continuous spiral round the breast starting at the clavicle.

The nipples should then be gently expressed for any discharge and tested with haemostix for the presence of blood if indicated.

Finally, the arm should be lowered and the axilla palpated for any lymph nodes.

The other breast should be examined in a similar way. The breasts should be held in the hands to assess any weight discrepancy between each breast.

Cervical smear screening

In the United Kingdom a comprehensive national screening programme for cervical cancer is in progress and the public are becoming more aware of the need for screening.

Family Practitioner Committees and General Practitioners have set up comprehensive call and re-call systems. The patient should be called up three-yearly if sexually active, with regular follow-up up to the age of 65 years.

Guidelines for taking cervical smears

Who should be screened?
    All women who are or have been sexually active
When should screening start?
    Within two years of becoming sexually active
When should screening stop?
    In women over 65 years who have had at least two recent negative smears and no history of doubtful or positive smears
    In women who have had a total hysterectomy which included removal of the cervix for a benign lesion.

Special risk groups

Certain groups are at special risk and may need more frequent screening. These are:

- those who have many or more than one sexual partners;
- those whose partners have many sexual partners;
- those on the contraceptive pill for five years or more;
- those who smoke;
- those with a history or presence of vaginal and/or vulval warts;
- those whose partners have or have had a history of penile or anal warts;
- those who have had a previous abnormal smear;
- those who have recently given birth, or had a miscarriage or abortion.

Method for taking smear

The smear itself is taken by scraping cells from the cervix uteri at the junction between the endocervix (columnar epithelium) and the ectocervix (squamous epithelium). It is at this transitional zone that carcinogenic changes may take place. It is important, therefore, to have scrapings of cells from both the endocervix and the ectocervix. Figure 9.2 shows the structure of the cervix in detail.

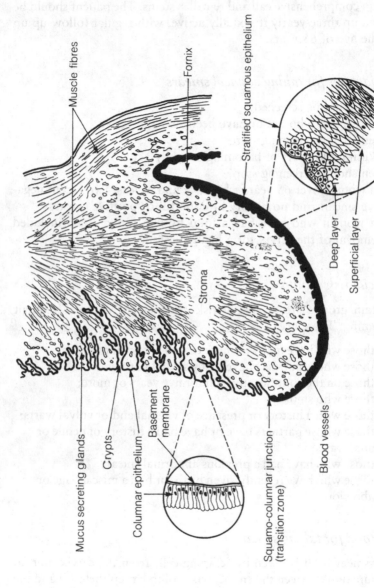

Figure 9.2 The structure of the cervix and the columnar–squamous junction.

Muscle fibres

Fornix

Stratified squamous epithelium

Deep layer

Superficial layer

Stroma

Blood vessels

Mucus secreting glands

Crypts

Columnar epithelium

Basement membrane

Squamo-columnar junction (transition zone)

The equipment needed for taking a smear is as follows:

- Vaginal speculum, either metal or plastic (disposable);
- Ayres spatula *or*
  Aylesbury spatula *or* } see notes below for instrument of choice
  Cytobrush;
- Glass slide;
- Fixative;
- Fixative slide container;
- Slidebox for transportation;
- Swab sticks and medicine;
- Sponge-holding forceps and cotton wool swabs;
- Request form;
- FP74 if appropriate for claiming (Figure 9.3);
- Pencil;
- Pathology request form;
- Latex gloves (the latter afford greatest protection since they are seam free);
- Clinical waste disposal means – for used disposables;
- Effective cleaning/sterilization of equipment – bearing in mind Department of Health guidelines.

The Aylesbury wooden disposable spatula gives a better sampling from the endocervical canal than the Ayres spatula.

The Cytobrush of which there are several types, is an excellent means of sampling the endocervical canal *but* an ectocervical smear is also necessary. The use of the cytobrush should be reserved for:

- Follow-up of patients who have received laser treatment for cervical lesions;
- Patients in whom an endocervical lesion is suspected;
- Postmenopausal women where the squamo-columnar junction has risen up into the cervical canal.

The procedure for taking the smear should be explained to the patient initially and at each step, with any questions answered as they arise.

The patient should have an empty bladder and be comfortable on the couch in the left lateral, lithotomy or recumbent position.

The labia, vulva and introitus should be examined and the warmed speculum inserted gently directed downwards; as the

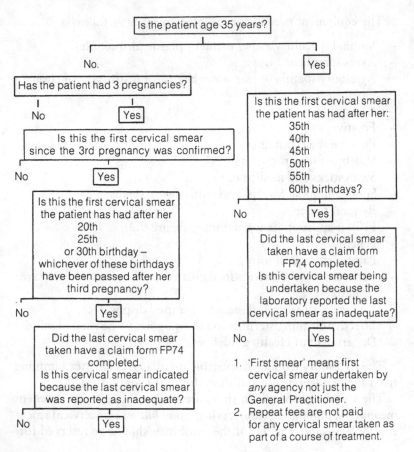

Figure 9.3 Guidelines for completion of claim form FP47.

speculum is gently and slowly inserted under good visualization and light, the walls of the vagina can be examined.

The speculum needs to be opened gently and manipulated until the cervix is clearly visible. The speculum blades should then be fixed open.

If any discharge is seen take a swab and, with sponge-holding forceps and a cotton wool swab, clean round the area of the cervix prior to taking the smear.

Take the spatula and place the leading tip in the cervical os, then rotate through 360° so that the other tip of the spatula scrapes the cervix (Figure 9.4). When a post-natal smear is being taken it may be appropriate to use the broad end of the spatula for taking the smear, or where there is evidence of erosion, scraping the cells beyond the erosion.

Spread the collected material thinly and evenly on a glass slide, moving the spatula in one direction on one side of the slide and then up the other side of the same slide. The slide should be clearly labelled in pencil with the patient's name, date of smear test and the patient's date of birth.

The slide should next be fixed and allowed to dry before being packed for transportation. Only remove the speculum if you are satisfied that the slide taken is satisfactory. Before removing the speculum, release the fixing of the opened speculum and remove gently, ensuring the vagina is not pinched as the instrument is removed.

Perform a vaginal examination to palpate the cervix, its mobility, the fornices, the deep pelvic areas and the coccyx and, bi-manually, the uterus, tubal and ovarian areas; ask the patient to press down to demonstrate any degree of prolapse tendency.

Wipe the introitus free of any lubricant and give the patient a clean paper towel with which to make herself comfortable. Allow privacy for the patient to get dressed.

Time should be given to explain to the patient how and when to expect a result.

Action for abnormal smears

If abnormal cells are found, the pathologist will request repeat smears at specific intervals or advise gynaecological referral.

Inadequate or unsatisfactory smears

A smear result will be reported as inadequate or unsatisfactory for the following reasons:

1. Scanty cell count
   If the cell count is insufficient, repeat the smear applying firm pressure to the squamo-columnar junction.
   If the cell count is insufficient because of atrophic vaginitis, a slightly moistened spatula may help.
2. Heavily blood stained smear
   Smear taken during menstruation should be avoided;

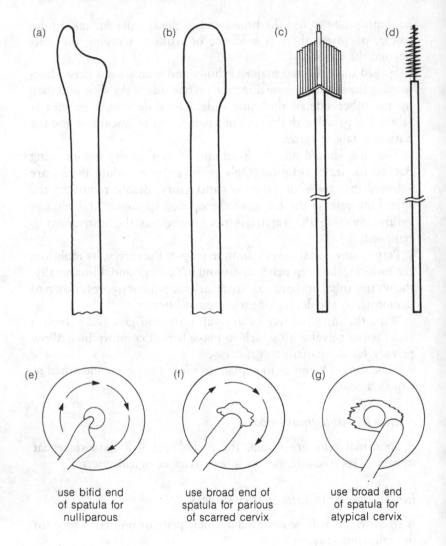

use bifid end
of spatula for
nulliparous

use broad end of
spatula for parious
of scarred cervix

use broad end
of spatula for
atypical cervix

Figure 9.4 Cervical smear instruments and technique; (a) Aylesbury spatula (bifid end of spatula); (b) broad end of Aylesbury spatula; (c) and (d) examples of cytobrushes. Use the appropriate end of the spatula and rotate through 360° in order to sample the whole of the columnar–squamous junction (transition zone); (e) use bifid end of spatula for nulliparous cervix, (f) use broad end of spatula for parous or scarred cervix; (g) use broad end of spatula for atypical cervix.

3. Epithelial content obscured by pus
   Where there is thick mucopurulent exudate present, remove this using a dry cotton wool swab on sponge-holding forceps before taking the smear. If indicated, take a high vaginal swab for pathology;
4. Air-dried smear
   The remedy for an air-dried smear is to apply the fixative immediately!

CLASSIFICATION OF CERVICAL SMEAR RESULTS

Recommended in the Report of the Intercollegiate Working Party on Cervical Cytology Screening (1987)

Cytology	Action
Unsatisfactory	Repeat
Negative	Routine recall at recommended interval
Doubtful or borderline changes	Treat any infection, repeat Smear in 3 months
Koilocytosis and other warty changes	Repeat Cervical Smear 6–12 months and manage according to results
Persistant abnormalities	Refer for Colposcopy

Positive Cervical Smear Results

Dyskaryosis

Dyskaryosis means abnormal nucleus. Dyskaryosis is used to describe nuclear abnormalities that are more numerous or severe than inflammation alone.

The term Dyskaryosis is used in many ways:
CIN 1; CIN 11; CIN 111 (CIN: Cervical Intraepithelial Neoplasia)

Mild dyskaryosis	Two normal smears required before returning to routine screening programme. If confirmed in second smear at 3–6 months refer for colposcopy*
Moderate dyskaryosis	Refer for Colposcopy/Gynaecology*
Severe dyskaryosis	Refer for Colposcopy/Gynaecology*

Mild Dyskaryosis

Mild dyskaryosis usually have plentiful, thin, translucent cytoplasm with angular borders, resembling superficial or intermediate squamous cells. The nucleus occupies less than half the total area of cytoplasm.

Mild dyskaryosis correlates with cells from CIN 1. It is doubtful, if it can be distinguished from the nuclear abnormalities associated with human papilloma virus infection.

Moderate dyskaryosis

These cells have more disproportionate nuclear enlargement than mildly dyskaryotic cells. The nucleus occupies one half to two thirds of the cytoplasm.

Severe dyskaryosis

These cells have a typically narrow rim of thick dense cytoplasm. They are round, oval, polygonal or elongated in shape. The abnormal nucleus practically fills the cell or at least two thirds of it. Severely dyskaryotic cells correlate with cells from the surface of the cervical epithelium showing CIN 111 or invasive carcinoma.

GIVING UP SMOKING CLINIC

The introduction of tobacco into England after its discovery by Sir Walter Raleigh in the 17th century has created enormous problems to all ages of the population.

---

* These classifications vary from District to District it is important, therefore, to determine how the 'cyto-pathologist reports cervical smear findings in your District.

Effects of cigarette smoking

Some 100 000 deaths per year in Britain are contributable to cigarette smoking.

Tobacco contains tar and nicotine and produces carbon monoxide. These products affect the body in different ways – raising the blood pressure and pulse rate, reducing appetite, making the cilia within the respiratory system less effective which results in an accumulation of tenacious mucus. Carbon monoxide competes with oxygen for the haemoglobin and thereby reduces oxygen transference to the tissues where it is vital for cell function and normal cell development. Carbon monoxide also causes vasoconstriction of blood vessels.

The main toxic constituents of tobacco

1. Nicotine	An alkaloid that affects the central nervous system, having a stimulating effect. Increases heart rate and cardiac output. This puts extra strain on the heart and coronary arteries, causing the arteries to go into spasm which results in a reduced lumen diameter;
2. Carbon monoxide	This has a higher affinity of binding to haemoglobin than does oxygen and thus acts to displace oxygen from the haemoglobin molecule, resulting in a reduction in the capacity of haemoglobin to carry oxygen of 15%;
3. Tar	This is the residue of smoke. It is a thick, tenacious substance which affects the cilia lining the respiratory system. Tar is thought to be a pre-cancerous stimulant;
4. Irritants	These are mainly responsible for chronic bronchitis. They stimulate the production of thick mucous which inhibits cilia action in the respiratory tract.

The patient is more prone, therefore, to suffer from:

- heart disease;
- hypertension;
- gastric ulcers;
- bronchitis;
- carcinoma of the mouth, trachea, lungs and bladder (this risk also applies to cigar and pipe smokers).

The facts about smoking are that of 1000 young male adults in England who smoke, one will be murdered, six will die from road accidents, and 250 will die prematurely due to the effects of smoking. Fifty percent of children under the age of 14 admit to smoking, and 34% of all adults in the United Kingdom smoke.

There is also a risk from passive smoking: where there is one member of the family who smokes 20 cigarettes or more a day, the remainder of the family are twice as likely to develop lung cancer compared with a family who are totally non-smokers.

The Giving Up Smoking Clinic

This is essentially a self-help group. Each member needs to be motivated and really want to give up smoking.

Small numbers are probably more effective, say approximately ten.

Attention needs to be given to the room, ventilation, comfort, health education leaflets, questionnaires and evaluation sheets.

The patient is invited to attend and an appointment is given. Detailed planning of timing to suit your target population is important.

The invitation may be by personal contact with a follow-up letter.

Identifying the patients

Patients who might benefit from a giving up smoking clinic can be identified by:

- Advertising through the usual channels within the Surgery
- An opportunistic approach when patients attend for consultation
- Contact in other health screening clinics undertake in the practice or health centre, such as:
  - Planned screening programmes for new patients;

- Family planning clinics;
- Ante-natal clinics;
- Post-natal clinics;
- Traveller's clinics;
- Child health clinics.

First meeting

The first meeting is a getting-to-know each other type of session. The aim of this is to try to reduce tension and help to facilitate a self-help group.

There may need to be discussion about smoking and its affects. The use of reinforcement literature should be done with discretion.

This is the time when each member enters into a contract with the convener of the group. The terms of the contract may need to be negotiated. It is important to sign the contract and to give a copy to the patient, with the convener keeping one.

Patients are also encouraged to keep a diary so they can decide what type of smoker they are. Patients can record their experience in the following categories:

- smoked because it was essential; could not do without it;
- smoked because it felt necessary;
- smoked but could have done without it;
- opened packet but did not smoke cigarette.

The aims of the course need to be decided upon and agreed by all the group.

The weeks that follow will be devoted to the group's needs, identifying where individuals are vulnerable, and getting the patient's family involved.

Self-help methods

The following list of self-help tips may be helpful to patients.

The first cigarette of the day
- have a drink by the bed;
- change the routine.

Tea or coffee break cigarette
- try fruit juice or bovril;

- occupy your hands by knitting or Rubik's cube;
- sit with non-smoking colleagues.

The stress cigarette
- try to relax;
- seek distraction.

The boredom cigarette
- do something to occupy hands;
- ask non-smokers what they do;
- eat a carrot and a stick of celery;
- stand in front of the mirror and say 'I am a non-smoker'.

The leisure cigarette
- try and keep busy;
- chew gum;
- eat an apple.

The reward cigarette
- buy something with the money saved;
- go out with the money saved.

The average packet of cigarettes costs approximately £1.80 per packet of 20. A person who smokes 20 a day will save £12.60 per week which is £54.60 per month or £655.20 per year.

Withdrawal symptoms

The following list of withdrawal symptoms can be produced by the group, duplicated and distributed to each member. How to help with each symptom can be self-determined and shared within the group.

- craving;
- irritability;
- headaches;
- lightheadedness and dizziness;
- sleeplessness;
- tiredness;
- sore tongue, mouth ulcers and gastric disorders.

Aids to giving up smoking

Hypnosis and acupuncture may help some people to give up smoking, but some patients revert to their original smoking habits.

Nicotine chewing gum, which can be used for months, seems to help some patients. It is expensive and can only be obtained from the General Practitioner by private prescription. This product is not available on the National Health Service, and the patient, therefore, has to pay the full price for the gum. The patient who uses this method needs to be clearly instructed about chewing the gum slowly, and should be monitored as to progress.

SETTING UP A DIABETIC PRACTICE CLINIC

Diabetes mellitus

This is a metabolic disease of unknown cause resulting from a deficiency of the pancreatic hormone insulin.

The condition was first documented by the Ancient Egyptians, but it was the Ancient Greeks who defined it and used the word 'diabetes', meaning to syphon, having noticed that 'fellows' who had the condition suffered from polyuria.

Later the Romans added 'mellitus' derived from the Latin word 'sweet' on their discovery of sugar content of the urine of sufferer.

There are two types of diabetes, (1) Insulin dependent diabetes, and (2) non-insulin dependent diabetes.

Insulin dependent diabetes

The insulin-secreting cells of the Islets of Langerhans in the pancreas have become completely destroyed, possibly as a result of an immune process. These patients are often young when diagnosed, and fairly thin, and need insulin injections to survive.

Insulin-dependent diabetics usually remain under the care of Diabetic Physician. Some General Practitioners, however, have a shared care arrangement for their patients with the hospital service.

Non-insulin dependent diabetes

The insulin-secreting cells of the Islets of Langerhans are normal, but either the insulin is decreased or it has a decreased sensitivity.

These patients are predominantly over the age of 45 years – in which case the condition is known as late-onset diabetes. Patients are often obese, do not need insulin to survive and may be controlled by diet or oral hypoglycaemics alone.

Causes, associated diseases and risk factors, current care

Genetic factors influence both insulin dependent and non-insulin dependent diabetics. The exact pattern of inheritance is as yet not known.

Diabetes mellitus may be caused by or affected by, other factors, such as hormonal effects in Cushing's Syndrome; a possible effect from steroids or the contraceptive pill has been suggested by some authorities and effects from pregnancy.

The disease is often associated with hypertension; ischaemic heart disease; hyperlipidaemia; hypothyroidism.

The following risk factors should be taken into account with patients suffering from diabetes mellitus: obesity; cigarette smoking; alcohol consumption.

The current trend in the care of diabetics is towards care outside the hospital for patients who are non-insulin dependent. Until relatively recently their care has been hospital-based. However, Diabetic Practice Clinics are now being established and run effectively in General Practice settings. Those who attend are non-insulin dependent. The insulin-dependent diabetics continue to be monitored principally by hospitals.

Setting up a diabetic (practice) clinic

The aims of running a diabetic clinic within general practice are:

- To monitor all patients with diabetes mellitus;
- To identify any complications early and treat them;
- To help patients understand diabetes and its treatment, thereby removing some of the anxiety and ignorance which still surrounds the condition. Informed knowledge should help the patient lead a healthier and symptom-free life.

It is important to involve all the practice staff. This helps the practice to run smoothly because the staff are able to handle any queries which may arise. It also allows their role in the new venture to be determined and in-service training given. Involvement is an important aspect in obtaining staff co-operation, and is a motivating factor in job satisfaction and performance.

The incidence of diabetes mellitus in General Practice is approximately 1–2% of patients.

Identification of patients

Patients with diabetes mellitus can be identified within a practice in the following ways:

- Their records should be coded using the RCGP Colour Code which is brown;
- Through the disease index in the age-sex register;
- Repeat prescription requests (ordering diabetic-type medication e.g. oral hypoglycaemic agents);
- From new patient history and health questionnaire;
- By computer search;
- Through self-identification in response to publicity on the practice noticeboard asking patients to make themselves known.

Informing the patient

Patients can be informed about the services of a diabetic clinic through information displayed on the practice noticeboard or in a practice leaflet or booklet.

The invitation letter

An invitation to attend the diabetic clinic should consist of a letter of explanation to the diabetic patient, with an appointment, i.e. date and time to attend. The letter should contain the following information as well:

1. The patient will be requested to have had a normal meal some two hours' prior to the appointment;
2. The patient should bring a specimen of urine passed prior to the meal;
3. The patient is also asked to bring a driving companion or to have arranged transport because of the use of mydratic eye drops. These drops dilate the pupil for fundi examination.

Personnel in attendance at the diabetic clinic

The following people should be available to run the clinic:

- The Family Doctor;
- The Practice Nurse;
- And/or the District Health Authority attached Nursing Sister;
- The Dietitian from the District Health Authority with special interest in diabetes;
- The Chiropodist.

It is recommended that patients should be seen every six months for the following:

- Blood sugar;
- Urine;
- Weight.

Patients should be seen annually for:

- Blood pressure;
- Urine for proteinuria;
- Fundi examination;
- General medical examination;
- Foot examination;
- Weight.

Investigations

Weight

This should be measured regularly at all visits. Weight gives a good indication of diabetic state since it reflects diet consumption – a very important aspect of the disease.

For obese patients the calorific content of their diet will need to be checked.

Blood pressure

This should be checked as necessary according to history and/or medication.

If indicated, an ECG should also be performed to look for damage, myocardial infarction or arrythmias.

Urine

Urine should be analysed for glucose using Diastix. Patients should be encouraged to check their urine twice daily and will be given charts to plot their results.

The patient may be visited at home to check on the result. Home testing in the elderly may be misleading as they often have a raised renal threshold.

If a trace of protein is found in the urine, the patient is asked to produce an MSU. If protein is present in the MSU then a specimen should be sent to the laboratory for microscopy and pathology and also for serum creatinine and protein levels which would suggest probable renal impairment or malfunction.

The presence of ketones in the urine is an indication to look closely at the patient's dietary habits, particularly content and quantities.

Skin care

Diabetic patients commonly suffer from skin rashes and infections, varicose ulcers and pruiritis vulvae, and all these aspects of care need to be carefully monitored.

The patient's feet and toenails should be inspected and, where necessary, chiropody follow-up appointments made. Detailed care of the feet needs to be emphasized to the patient – the use of a video demonstrating foot care may help.

Eyes

Visual accuity should be checked. The patient will have homatrophine drops instilled prior to detailed examination of the fundi by the Doctor.

If there is any deviation from normal, the patient must be referred to an Ophthalmologist for an opinion.

Blood

Interpretation of blood sugar levels:

1–2 mmol/l = low;
4–10 mmol/l = ideal;
13 mmol/l or above = high.

Measurement of glycosylated HbA — this gives a better index of diabetic control, especially for the insulin-dependent diabetic. Also useful measurement for patient compliance for the patient controlled by diet or hypoglycaemic drugs.

A check should be made for raised levels of cholesterol in the blood, and also for any electrolyte imbalance.

General medical examination

Carried out on an annual basis, this should include checking peripheral pulses.

Diet

This is the fundamental aspect of care of the non-insulin dependent diabetic patient. The dietitian, both individually and possibly on a group basis, will be able to offer dietary advice and can at the same time check the patient's compliance.

The Diabetic Association publishes a set of dietary recommendations from time to time. Currently, it is recommended that the carbohydrate content should contain more high fibre foods such as beans, cereals and wholemeal bread. Less animal fat should be consumed, chicken or fish should be encouraged and skimmed milk and low cholesterol oils and spreads used.

Many elderly non-insulin dependent diabetic patients find strict adherence to a sugar-free diet almost impossible, and the fact that a digestive or rich tea biscuit as a substitute can be taken often cheers them!

Hypoglycaemic drugs

When dietary management alone does not control diabetes, oral hypoglycaemic drugs become a necessary form of control. They fall into two groups: (1) the sulphonylureas; (2) the bogonides.

The sulphonylureas

These are principally given to non-insulin dependent diabetics who are non-obese, and they are long acting hypoglycaemia agents.

These drugs are contraindicated in: pregnancy; in patients under 40 years; and in patients with a past history of Ketosis.

The sulphonylureas include:

- Tolbutamide;
- Chlorpropamide (Diabenese) – long acting up to 60 hours;
- Glibenclamide;
- Glibenese;
- Diamicron.

The following side-effects of these drugs have been noted:

- can cause gastro-intestinal upsets;
- skin rashes may develop;
- alcohol, Aspirin and Tagamet can prolong hypoglycaemic effect;
- Septrin or Bactrin can prolong the action.

The Bigonides

These are principally given to obese patients and are used as additional treatment when the sulphonylureas are not totally effective. They have a short action time of approximately 8–12 hours.

General advice and health education

The autonomic nervous system is often affected by diabetes, causing disorders of the bowel bladder and also impotence for which the patient will need counselling.

Alcohol consumption and smoking habits will need to be discussed, and appropriate advice given.

Exercise is a vital aspect of care and regular exercise needs to be encouraged for the diabetic patient's continued well being.

The patient will also need regular medical examinations for fitness to drive.

Diabetic patients are exempt from prescription charges and they will need to complete the appropriate DHSS form.

A number of videos are available for the patient with diabetes, either through pharmaceutical firms or through the local Health Education Office.

A variety of booklets are available from the British Diabetic Association at: 10 Queen Anne Street, London W1M 0BD.

PRE-CONCEPTUAL CARE OR PRE-PREGNANCY HEALTH

It is recognized that the health of both parents at the time of conception is as important as the health of the expectant mother during pregnancy. Preparation for parenthood begins, therefore, before the baby is conceived.

There are some environmental factors, however, that whilst affecting an individual cannot be changed, such as pollution.

Peri-natal mortality and morbidity rates have reduced, but these rates can still be improved. It is anticipated that pre-conceptual care will help in their reduction.

There are a number of factors which are know to affect the outcome of pregnancy:

— Maternal age;
— Parity;
— Socio-economic status of the father of the baby;
— Maternal health.

Pre-conceptual care is a means, whether such care is given on an *ad hoc* basis for example at a Family Planning Clinic or at Pre-Conceptual Care Clinics, of identifying problems, and referring where appropriate. The Practice Nurse in this situation is a health educator, a resource person and also uses her/his skills to identify problems.

Medical aspects of pre-conceptual care

• Blood test for Rubella status;
• Blood pressure;
• Weight;
• Height;
• Urine analysis;
• Blood profile;
• Cervical smear.

Details of the health of both partners

• General health;
• Life style;
• Contraception;
• Eating habits.

The above information provides a baseline from which to assess changes during pregnancy.

Nutrition

Detailed information about what is eaten and how the food is cooked may highlight areas which need to be improved. The couple can motivate each other in the important area of nutrition.

Advice should be aimed at improving the diet of the couple but it should be adapted to suit individuals and their own particular life-style.

The following given a brief description of the main nutritional requirements:

1. Protein	Sources of amino acids for growth and repair. They can also be converted into carbohydrate, providing an alternative source of energy;
2. Carbohydrate	As a source of glucose for ATP production or for storage of glycogen;
3. Fat	A concentrated source of energy and essential fatty acids and fat-soluble vitamins (A,D,E,K);
4. Vitamins	Fat soluble A,D,E,K Water Soluble thiamin, riboflavin, niacin, pyridoxine, ascorbic acid, folic acid, cobalamin – responsible for forming co-enzymes which control normal growth and development;
5. Minerals	Calcium, phosphorus, sulphur, potassium, sodium, chlorine, magnesium, iron, fluorine, zinc, copper, iodine, manganese, chromium, cobalt; – regulate pH of body fluids and regulate all body processes. Compose bone and teeth;
6. Water	Composes two-thirds of body weight, essential for life.

Figure 9.5 summarizes the various socio-economic factors that can influence an individual's dietary intake. In summary, implementing a programme of good eating involves the following:

1. Provision of advice and guidelines;
2. Implementing these guidelines effectively.

Complex dietary requirements of a couple or individual may need specialist help from a Nutritionalist or a Counsellor.

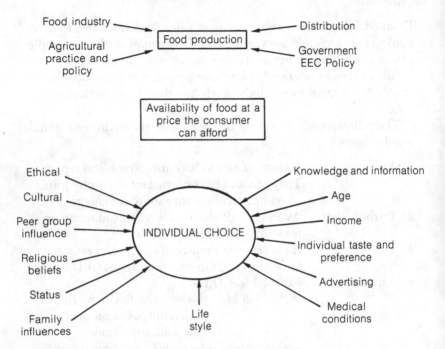

Figure 9.5 Influences on food consumption.

Weight

In order to establish the correct weight for a patient, their height needs to be determined, followed by use of the weight/height chart and discussion of the findings with the patient.

Patients who conceive when they are overweight are at greater risk of developing complications in pregnancy and childbirth.

Patients who are considerably underweight for their height may be temporarily infertile and may have menstrual irregularities.

Rubella status

Rubella (German measles) is a very mild infectious illness which patients very often suffer from without even knowing they are doing so. The symptoms and signs, which may last only a few days, may be those of a mild rash, slight fever, swollen glands, and aching joints.

The rubella virus is particularly dangerous to those patients who are pregnant in the early stages of embryonic and fetal development (the first 12 weeks of pregnancy). All systems of the developing fetus may be affected, causing such abnormalities as deafness, blindness, or cardiac anomalies.

Rubella immunization is now offered to all schoolgirls from 10 years of age. This immunization does not guarantee lifetime immunity and rubella status is determined in all patients who attend for ante-natal care, irrespective of whether the patient has previously been immunized or not. If the patient is found not to have rubella antibodies, immunization is offered during the post-natal period.

With concentrated pre-conceptual care, of course, patients will have their rubella status determined prior to conceiving. Patients immunized in adulthood should be advised to avoid becoming pregnant for some three months after rubella immunization.

Measles, mumps and rubella immunization is now available for those babies who would between the ages of 15 months and 2 years be having measles immunization, and for children prior to going to school.

Contraception

Discussion with regard to family planning will focus upon the couple's plan for starting a family.

In order to establish the expected date of delivery with any degree of accuracy those women who have been taking the contraceptive pill should be advised to stop taking it some three months before contemplating pregnancy, by which time the patient's menstrual cycle should have returned to normal. During this three-month period alternative methods of contraception, such as the barrier methods, will need to be discussed.

Patients with an intra-uterine device *in situ* will need to have this removed if they want to start a family.

Smoking

Smoking adversely affects an individual and others in many ways. The woman or her partner who smoke are putting not only themselves at risk but also the embryo/fetus should they continue to smoke during pregnancy.

There is an increased risk of spontaneous abortion, fetal-growth retardation, retardation of intellectual development, fetal abnormalities, and a higher risk of perinatal mortality since smoking may cause placenta abruptio.

It is known that carbon monoxide reduces the oxygen-carrying ability of haemoglobin, so the supply of oxygen to the fetus is reduced. Oxygen supply and nutrients necessary for normal growth may be also reduced since smoking may cause the arterioles to go into spasm, preventing exchange of these substances across the placenta. Nicotine inhibits the action of the breathing movements of the fetus *in utero*, and a baby once born may suffer from respiratory distress.

Therefore, if one or both partners smoke, they should be strongly advised and supported to give up smoking before contemplating pregnancy.

Alcohol

Fetal Alcohol Syndrome is sadly a reality and results from an expectant mother drinking alcohol to excess during pregnancy. The fetus *in utero* is often hyperactive, small for dates and is born with characteristic facies, which are often associated with abnormalities of heart, limbs and central nervous system. The baby demonstrates all the signs of alcohol withdrawal.

Any excess the expectant mother takes in pregnancy which is not detoxicated in her liver will readily pass through the placenta to the fetus, resulting in the syndrome described.

The drinking habits of both partners should be reviewed as part of pre-conceptual care, and appropriate support given.

Medicines and drugs

Any patient needing long-term medication for such problems as hypertension, epilepsy, diabetes, asthma and cardiac conditions will need expert advice and support from a specialist.

Those patients who are addicted to some form of controlled drug will also need specialist care.

Exercise

The couple who are planning to start a family should also be encouraged to take some form of exercise unless there is a medical problem which contraindicates this.

The publication, *Exercise – Why Bother?* produced by the Sports Council provides a simple guide to getting fitter for adults of all ages.

Emotional support

This kind of support from a Practice Nurse can be very valuable and it will vary from couple to couple or individual to individual as relationships are formed and different topics are discussed.

Work environment

The type of work the patient who is planning for her pregnancy currently undertakes should be determined and any help or advice given.

If specific advice is needed, such as working with VDUs or in an area where smoking takes place, the health and safety representative at a place of work should be able to advise, as should the Family Doctor.

Social conditions

Anxiety arising from poor social conditions, social isolation, or inadequate funds can perhaps be helped in a practical way, particularly by support from the Health Visitor.

Claim for maternity benefit

The conditions for Maternity Allowance and Maternity Grant are explained in the Leaflet NI 17A which can be obtained from the patient's local social security office.

Other financial support can also be discussed at the patient's local social security office, although the Midwife and Health visitor may be able to give immediate advice.

Table 9.1 *Alcohol contents of drink*

Beverage		Grams of alcohol	Units of alcohol
Beers and lagers	ordinary strength (3% alcohol)	8g/½ pint	1.0
		12g/can	1.5
		16g/pint	2.0
	export beer (4% alcohol)	16g/can	2.0
		20g/pint	2.5
	strong beer or lager (5.5% alcohol)	16g/½ pint	2.0
		24g/can	3.0
		32g/pint	4.0
	extra strength beer or lager (7% alcohol)	20g/½ pint	2.5
		32g/can	4.0
		40g/pint	5.0
Ciders	average cider (4% alcohol)	12g/½ pint	1.5
		24g/pint	3.0
	strong cider (6% alcohol)	16g/½ pint	2.0
		32g/pint	4.0
		64/quart bottle	8.0
Spirits	whisky 70 proof (40% alcohol)	8g/single measure in England and Wales	1.0
	brandy 70 proof (40% alcohol)	12g/single measure in Scotland and N. Ireland	1.5
	whisky, gin, vodka (40% alcohol)	240g/bottle	30.0
Table wines	table wines (10% alcohol)	8g/standard glass	1.0
		56g/bottle	7.0
		100g/litre bottle	12.5

Table 9.1 *Cont.*

Beverage		Grams of alcohol	Units of alcohol
Fortified wine	sherry port vermouth (20% alcohol)	8g/standard measure 120g/bottle	1.0 15.0
liquers	liquers (20% alcohol)	8g/small measure 100–240g/bottle	1.0 12.5–30.0

Outside support

Several organizations are committed to pre-conceptual care:

- Health Education Council;
- Family Planning Association;
- Spastics Society;
- Maternity Alliance;
- Foresight.

THE PATIENT WITH AN ALCOHOL PROBLEM

The consumption of alcohol is measured according to standard units. Half pint of beer, a glass of wine, sherry or single measure of spirits are equivalent to one unit (Figure 9.4). A detailed breakdown of the alcohol content of drinks is given in Table 9.1.

Most individuals are very sensitive about their alcohol intake but in screening programmes for men (MOT) and women it is now a routine measure to ask about alcohol consumption.

Environment and culture play an important role in an individual's drinking behaviour. There is increasing concern about the Asian community and other immigrants to this country, many of whom are becoming dependent drinkers.

It remains a fact that men consume more alcohol than women, but this pattern is gradually changing.

Acceptable levels of alcohol consumption are as follows:

- Men – up to 21 units a week spread throughout the week;
- Women – up to 14 units a week spread throughout the week.

Figure 9.7 shows how quickly the effects wear off.

Effects of alcohol abuse

Central nervous system

- Blackouts

Neuropsychiatric

- Insomnia;
- Anxiety;
- Depression;
- Suicide;
- Amnesia.

Nerves

- Weakness;
- Paraesthesiae of hands – Karsakoff Syndrome.

Cerebrovascular

- Cerebral vascular accidents;
- Subarachnoid haemorrhage;
- Subdural haematoma.

Liver

- Fatty infiltration of liver;
- Hepatitis;
- Cirrhosis;
- Liver failure.

Gastro-intestinal

- Reflux oesophagitis;
- Gastritis;
- Diarrhoea;

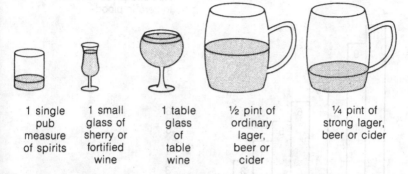

Figure 9.6 Amounts of different drinks which are equivalent to one unit when measuring alcohol consumption.

- Impaired absorption of food;
- Chronic pancreatitis;
- Weight loss due to toxic affects of alcohol;
- Obesity in the early stages.

Cardiovascular system

- Palpitations;
- Chronic heart failure.

Respiratory system

- Bronchitis;
- Pneumonia from inhalation of vomit.

Muscular and skeletal systems

- Muscle weakness;
- Myopathy;
- Gout.

Reproductive system

- Loss of libido;
- Impotence;

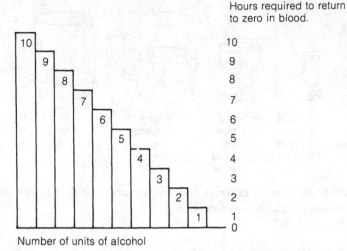

Figure 9.7 The number of hours required for blood level of alcohol to return to zero.

- Sexual difficulties;
- Menstrual irregularities.

Social

- Family fighting and violence;
- Absenteeism from college, school or work;
- Repeated arguments;
- Aggression;
- Divorce.

Legal problems

- Accidents at work; home; sea; on the roads;
- Breach of the peace;
- Vagrancy;
- Drinking and driving;
- Assault;

- Homicide;
- Manslaughter.

Work

- Absenteeism;
- Accidents;
- Poor performance;
- Poor leadership.

Driving

- Alcohol is associated with one quarter of all road accidents;
- In fatal accidents occurring between 18–24 years of age, alcohol is the major cause.

Drug interactions

Alcohol may affect the action of certain drugs either by diminishing or enhancing their effect. The following drugs are affected by alcohol:

- Benzodiazepines;
- Barbiturates;
- Phenothiazines;
- Oral hypoglycaemic agents;
- Phenytoin;
- Warfarin;
- Monoamine oxidase inhibitors;
- Paracetamol.

Identifying the patient

Medical history

Any of the following may indicate alcohol abuse:

- Dyspepsia;
- Gastritis;
- Diarrhoea;
- Anxiety;

- Depression;
- Family disharmony;
- Liver disease;
- Frequent consultations;
- Tranquilizers;
- Hypertension;
- Casualty attendance letters indicating alcohol abuse.

Patient's present situation

- Indigestion;
- Nausea;
- Diarrhoea;
- Insomnia;
- Restlessness;
- Loss of interest;
- Depression;
- Financial problems;
- Problems with the law;
- Accidents;
- Trembling and lack of co-ordination – dropping items;
- Frequent outbursts at home and disharmony.

Alcohol consumption history

- Consumption over the last month;
- Consumption over the last week;
- Reason for starting to drink;
- Whether attempts have been made to stop drinking and what the outcome was.

Results from physical examination

- Plethoric and bloated face;
- Smell of alcohol;
- Bloodshot eyes;
- Poor oral hygiene;
- Tremor;
- Hypertension.

Investigations

No individual test for alcohol is a guaranteed indicator of alcohol abuse since results may be abnormal for reasons of disease. The most likely tests to give a positive result which is probably due to alcohol abuse are:

- Serum enzyme gammaglutamyl transferase (GGT);
- Red cell mean corpuscular volume (MCV).

The following results from other tests would support the above in indicating likely alcohol abuse:

- Raised serum urate;
- Raised fasting triglycerides;
- Raised aspartate aminotransferase.

The Alcometer test is used by the police and gives an accurate reading. The acceptable level of alcohol for driving is less than 35 micrograms of alcohol per 100 ml of breath.

Management

The following are general pointers for management of alcohol abuse.

Aim initially at short-term goals

- Ask the patients to keep a diary of alcohol consumption;
- Involve the patient's nearest relative or friend to give support and encouragement;
- Teach relaxation techniques;
- Review progress regularly;
- Do not regard relapse as a failure.

The patient may need to be referred by the doctor to a specialist unit. Support for the spouse and family of a patient suffering from alcoholism should not be overlooked.

It needs to be remembered that the elderly very often have an alcohol problem. This may be indicated by:

- Withdrawal symptoms;
- Fits or DTs;
- Neurosis or psychosis;
- Need for help in re-planning life;

- Peripheral neuropathy;
- Cirrhosis of the liver.

TRAVELLING ABROAD

The numbers of people travelling abroad, whether for package tours, service overseas, short trips or to stay for many years has increased considerably.

Nowadays, experienced travellers abroad tend to have fewer health problems. Preventative immunization programmes and advice for preventing ill health play their part in this.

Traveller abroad clinic

First consultation

This consultation should provide information about medical services abroad.

Leaflet SA40 issued by the Department of Health describes the free or reduced cost of medical treatments abroad. It also gives details about Form E111 which will cover for free or reduced cost of medical treatment when going to another European Community country.

Form E112 will need to be completed in the event of the patient seeking by intent medical treatment or maternity care abroad. Authorization has to be given by the Department of Health for this form to be issued.

The traveller should have with him/her: Passport; NHS Medical Card; Form E111; and possibly Form E112.

The Department of Health leaflet SA41 issues information on health protection whilst abroad.

In order to advise the patient, it is essential to find out all the countries to be visited, and in what order, also length of stay, mode of travel and life-style, and immunization history.

Second consultation

A return consultation 4−6 weeks later should meet the traveller's needs, although if primary courses are being given more visits will be required. Oral poliomyelitis vaccine should not be given at the same time as immunoglobulin.

Immunization programmes

Travellers are at increased risk from:

- Unfamiliar organisms;
- New strains of familiar organisms;
- Contaminated food and water;
- Insect bites;
- Intimate human contact.

Immunizations may be classified as being: (1) Compulsory: where evidence of vaccination is necessary before a traveller may enter the country; (2) Strongly advised; or (3) Recommended.

Compulsory immunizations

1. Yellow fever

Yellow fever is caused by a virus which is endemic in tropical forest areas. It mainly infects monkeys, but if travellers visit these areas then the virus may be transmitted via the mosquito, whose normal hosts are the monkeys. Immunization in Great Britain is undertaken at certain yellow fever vaccination centres. Details of the immunization are as follows:

- Live attenuated virus is used;
- 0.5 ml is given subcutaneously;
- The certificate is valid for 10 years, 10 days after vaccination;
- A boost is needed every 10 years.

The immunization is not recommended for patients who are:

- Pregnant;
- Immunosuppressant;
- Hypersensitive;
- Babies 9 months old and younger.

Immunizations which are strongly advised

1. Typhoid fever

Typhoid Fever is endemic worldwide. Spread is usually faecal-oral. The risks are increased where there are poor hygienic facilities. Details of the immunization are as follows:

- Heat killed *Salmonella typhi* is used;
- Patients over 10 years of age are given 0.5 ml subcutaneously or intramuscularly;
- This dose is repeated 4–6 weeks later;
- A booster required every three years.

The immunization is not recommended for children under one year of age.

2. Poliomyelitis

It is important to produce antibodies to all three serotypes of poliovirus. The immunization procedure is as follows:

- Live attenuated virus (3 serotypes) is used;
- 3 drops are given orally;
- The primary course consists of three immunizations at four-weekly intervals;
- A booster dose is needed every 10 years.

Poliomyelitis immunization is not recommended for patients who are:

- Pregnant;
- Immunosuppressed.

Poliomyelitis should not be given at the same time as immunoglobulin.

3. Tetanus

All individuals should receive an initial course or have had boosters to maintain immunity to tetanus. Immunization details are as follows:

- Inactivated toxin is used;
- 0.5 ml is given subcutaneously or intramuscularly;
- A 6 week interval is needed before the second dose if a primary course;
- A 6 month interval is needed between second and third doses if a primary course;
- A booster is needed every 5–10 years.

4. Cholera

Although cholera vaccination is recommended for those travelling in areas where this endemic, it must be recognized that cholera vaccination is of little value. The vaccination details are:

- Heat killed *Vibrio cholerae* is used;
- For patients over 10 years of age, 0.5 ml is given subcutaneously or intramuscularly;
- 4–6 weeks later 1.0 ml is given subcutaneously;
- For patients under 10 years, see manufacturer's instructions;
- The certificate of vaccination is valid for 6 months, 6 days after vaccination;
- A booster dose is needed every 6 months.

The immunization is not recommended for babies six months and under.

5. Hepatitis A

Hepatitis A is endemic worldwide, and is spread by the faecal-oral route. Hepatitis A antibody can be tested for. The presence of life-long immunity means immunoglobulin is not necessary.

If antibody is not present, immunoglobulin should be given just before departure; immunoglobulin can be given to children using reduced doses. The immunization details are:

- Concentrate of pooled human immunoglobulin is used;
- Adults given 250 mg intramuscularly are protected for 6 weeks;
- 500–750 mg given intramuscularly will protect an adult for approximately 6 months.

Malaria

Malaria is widespread in tropical and subtropical countries and is spread by the bite of a female anopheline mosquito that has been infected by the malaria parasite.

The increasing mobility of the population brings a further risk since travellers may be bitten by mosquitoes at airports *en route* as well as in the countries where they are staying. This means, of course, that the first symptoms may occur in a country where the disease would not normally be considered. Mosquitoes may also be brought into aeroplanes thus possibly infecting airport staff and other travellers.

Spread also occurs through the sharing of needles by drug addicts.

Determining the most appropriate drug for a particular traveller is not straightforward. The prevalence of the disease and the resistance to anti-malaria drugs is constantly changing. The public and the General Practitioner can obtain information from specialist centres. In some practices there is a direct link to these specialist centres through a computer.

Patients should therefore be advised to take the following personal precautions against malaria.

1. Avoid mosquito bites, especially after sunset when the anopheline mosquitoes responsible for transmitting malaria are most active. Long trousers, long sleeves, dresses, windows netted and mosquito nets over beds all help to prevent mosquito bites;
2. Start anti-malaria tablets at least one week before departure, not only to check on tolerance but also to build up blood concentrations before exposure.

Information about anti-malaria drugs

Fansidar, Maloprim, Chlorquine, Proguanil and Pyrimethamine rarely cause side-effects when given in the correct dose for malaria prophylaxis. Nausea may be prevented by advising the patient to take the tablets after a meal. Rashes may occur due to Maloprim as there is sulphone in the drug which is a sulphonamide derivative and this drug is not recommended for those patients who have a sensitivity to Sulphonamides. Prolonged used of Chloroquine may result in retinal changes. Progunil and Pyrimethamine may, rarely, cause haemopoietic problems. Supplementary doses of folic acid can be given.

The risks to the mother and the fetus during pregnancy outweigh prophylactic medication. Fansidar should be avoided during the last trimester and in the neonate (through breast milk). It is possible that this drug can cause jaundice by displacing unconjugated bilirubin from protein binding sites.

Parasites may persist in the liver and produce illness once the prophylaxis has stopped. Prophylaxis may also fail because the patient may not have taken the tablets regularly or in the correct dose, or gastro-intestinal upset may have resulted in the tablets not being absorbed.

Other advise

People planning to travel abroad should be given routine advice on the following subjects:

- Sun and heat;
- Altitude;
- Drinking water;
- Swimming;
- Personal hygiene;
- Food and alcohol;
- Skin care, bites and stings;
- Travelling with young children.

Patients with any of the following problems or conditions should also be given advice on whether to travel and how to cope overseas:

- Emotional and psychiatric problems;
- Heart disease;
- Pregnancy;
- Diabetes mellitus;
- Respiratory disorders;
- Long-term medication such as steroids.

AIDS

AIDS is caused by a virus known as the human immunodeficiency virus abbreviated to HIV. In France it is known LAV – Lymphadenopathy associated virus, and in America as HTLV-III – human T-cell leukaemia virus. The HIV virus is believed to be from a family of retroviruses which were unknown in humans before the 1980s but which have been linked with leukaemia-type illnesses in animals. HIV can reproduce itself only by invading a living cell, adapting it, and using its host to reproduce.

The cells in the human body which the virus attacks are known as T-helper cells (T4). These are specifically designed to aid the immune system of the body. The virus enters the cell and alters the DNA (Figure 9.8). The cell cannot then interpret the messages sent by the immune system as the virus places its own 'blueprint' onto that of the invaded cell, leaving the immune system deficient and enabling the virus to reproduce itself.

The virus can remain undetected in the body without obvious signs of infection. Some specific illnesses peculiar to HIV infection can present. The two most widely recognized as being indicative of full blown AIDS are:

- Pneumocystis carnii pneumonia (PCP);
- Kaposi's sarcoma.

Human immunodeficiency virus has been found in certain body fluids:

- Blood;
- Semen;
- Vaginal and cervical secretions;
- Saliva;
- Breast milk.

General symptons of HIV infection and AIDS

- Fatigue lasting weeks with no obvious cause;
- Unexplained weight loss over a short period of time;
- Lymphadenopathy;
- Oral candiasis;
- Rashes – fungal infections;
- Persistant diarrhoea;
- Night sweats and chills;
- Cytomegalovirus, retinitis, and pneumonitis;
- Hepatosplenomegaly;
- Frequent infections.

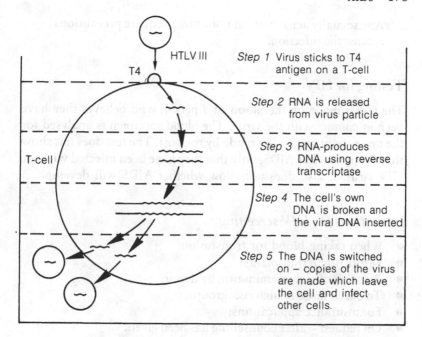

Figure 9.8 The infection of a T-cell by HTLV III. The HTLV-III virus infects cells. It is most likely to attack a T-cell. It actually attacks the T-cell by sticking to a special receptor on the surface called the T4 antigen. The T-cell uses this receptor to carry out specific tasks. It is considered that the T-cell mistakes the virus for something else and so lets it in or that the virus has adapted to this receptor. Once inside the cell, the virus rapidly sheds its coat.

Inside the virus, when it has lost its coat, is a single strand of RNA. The RNA builds a double-stranded section of DNA, inserts this DNA into the DNA of the cell, takes over the cell and starts making copies of the virus. In order for RNA to make DNA the virus has to produce a special chemical reverse transcriptase (RNA – dependent DNA polymerase) Nowhere else in the body or in other animals or mammals or circumstances is reverse transcriptase produced.

High risk groups

- Homosexual or bisexual men;
- Intravenous drug users;
- Haemophiliacs treated with blood products not treated for HIV;

— Any sexually active person not using adequate precautions against the infection.

Testing for HIV

The test is made on the blood of a person who believes they have been in contact with the virus. The blood specimen is analysed for the presence of antibodies made by the host. The test does not show that the person has AIDS, only that they have been infected with the HIV virus. It also does not show whether AIDS will develop.

Indications for HIV screening

- When taking blood for transfusion;
- Before organ transplants;
- Before artificial insemination by donor;
- To check those in high risk groups;
- For insurance applications;
- On request — after counselling has been given.

Where to obtain the test

Testing for HIV can be done by the General Practitioner; at a sexually transmitted disease clinic (special clinic); or by a genito-urinary clinic.

Informed consent, confidentiality and counselling

Of major importance for anybody being tested for HIV is the assurance of confidentiality of the test and results.

Informed consent implies that the reasons why the test is being advised are being carefully explained to the individual and that the results will also be carefully discussed.

Patients need to be counselled prior to and following testing by an experienced counsellor.

Many District Health Authorities are employing AIDS counsellors or co-ordinators, not only to be involved with and help in patient care, but also to fulfil an educational role for health personnel.

FURTHER READING

Well woman

Breast Cancer Screening (1986) Working Group Report. Prof. G.R. Patrick
Forrest, HMSO, London.

Roberts, H. (1981) *Women, Health and Reproduction*. Routledge and
Keegan Paul, London.

Lloyd, G. (1975) *Cervical Cytology Screening in General Practice*,
Churchill, Livingstone, Edinburgh.

McPherson, A.M. (1985) *Cervical Screening – A Practical Guide*, Oxford
Medical Publications.

Useful addresses

A Guide to Examining your Breast (leaflet)
The Health Education Council
78 New Oxford Street
London WC1A 1AH

The Abnormal Smear
The British Society for Colposcopy and Cervical
Pathology

Women's National Cancer Control Campaign
1 South Audley Street,
London W1Y 5DQ

Aylesbury Spatulae
Histopath Limited
Telephone: 0442 55446

The Jarvis Screening Centre
Stoughton Road
Guildford
Surrey
GU1 1LJ

Women's Health Information Centre
(for leaflet on *An Abnormal Smear: What does it mean?*)
52 Featherstone Street
London EC1

Smoking

ASH (1985) *Smoking Prevention – A Health Promotion Guide for the
NHS*. Handbook, London.

Stoppard, M. (1985) *Quit Smoking*, BBC Publications, London.

So you want to stop Smoking (Ref: AS33)
The Health Education Authority,
78 New Oxford Street,
London, WC1A 1AH.

The smoker's guide to non-smoking (Ref: AS23)
(Helping you to better health series)
The Health Education Authority,
78 New Oxford Street,
London, WC1A 1AH.

Useful addresses

Health Education Authority,
78 New Oxford Street,
London, WC1A 1AH.

ASH (Action on Smoking and Health)
Markgaret Pyke House,
5–11 Mortimer Street,
London, W1N 7RH.

Diabetes

Non-insulin dependent diabetics
Dr John Day
Thorsons, Wellington, New York.
(Available from British Diabetic Association)

Pre-conceptual care

Chamberlain, G. (1986) *Pre-Pregnancy Care: A Manual for Practice*,
    Wiley, Oxford.

Alcohol

Useful information for the family and friends of problem drinkers

Al-Anon Family Groups
61 Great Dover Street
London, SE1 4YF.

Alateen – Support for young people and teenagers who are affected by their family.

Both Al-Anon and Alateen may be contacted by the following telephone numbers:
London: Tel. 01 403 0888 (24 hour telephone service)
Belfast: Tel. 0232 243489
Glasgow: Tel. 041 221 7356
People living in Wales should telephone the London number.

Alcohol Concern Wales, 24 Park Place, Cardiff CF1 3BA
Tel. 0222 398791 378855

Scottish Council on Alcohol, 137–145 Sauchiehall Street, Glasgow G2 3EW.
Tel. 041 333 9677

Northern Ireland Council on Alcohol, 40 Elmwood Avenue, Belfast BT9 6AZ.
Tel. 0232 664434

For advice, information and access to a national network of over 40 local centres

Alcohol Concern,
305 Grays Inn Road,
London, WC1X 8QF.

For advice, information and counselling

The Accept Clinic,
200 Seagrave Road,
London, SW16 1RQ.
Tel. 01 381 3155/6

Let's Drink to your Health!
The British Psychological Society,
The Distribution Centre,
Blackhorse Road,
Letchworth,
Hertfordshire, SG6 1HN.

National Council on Alcoholism and the Medical
Council on Alcoholism,
3 Grosvenor Crescent,
London, SE1 4YF.

Health Education Authority,
78, New Oxford Street,
London, WC1A 1AH.
Tel. 01 631 0930
(Provides information and lists the local Health Education Departments.)

Foreign travel

Useful address

DHSS Leaflets Unit
Stanmore,
Middlesex, HA7 1AY.

Centres specializing in giving up to date medical advice for those persons intending to travel abroad

Department of Health and Social Security,
Alexander Fleming House,
Elephant and Castle,
London, SE1 6BY.

Hospital for Tropical Diseases,
4 St Pancras Way,
London, NW1 OPE.

Yellow fever vaccination centres

England and Wales

Yellow Fever Clinic,
Clinic 10,
Addenbrooke's Hospital
Hills Road,
Cambridge.

Yellow Fever Vaccination Service
Hospital for Tropical Diseases,
4 St Pancras Way,
London, NW1 OPE.

School of Tropical Medicine,
Pembroke Place,
Liverpool, L3 5QA.

Scotland

Central Vaccination Clinic,
9 St Johnston Terrace,
Edinburgh, EH1 2PP.

Northern Ireland

Yellow Fever Vaccination Centre,
Lincoln Avenue Clinic,
Antrim Road,
Belfast, BT14 6AZ.

Inactivated poliomyelitis vaccine available from

England	01 636 6811 X 3117
N. Ireland	0232 224431 X 330
Scotland	031 552 6255 X 2162
Wales	0222 825111 X 4658

Advice for patients who are handicapped in some way

Air Transport Users Committee,
129 Kingsway,
London, WC2B 6NN.

British Airways Medical Service,
Central Area Medical Unit,
Heathrow Airport,
Hounslow,
Middlesex.

British Diabetic Association,
10 Queen Anne Street,
London, W1M OBD.

National Association for Maternal and Child Welfare,
1 South Audley Street,
London, W1Y 6JS.

Medic-Alert Foundation,
11–13 Clifton Terrace,
London, N4 3JP.

AIDS

Sources of further information

Health Education Authority
78 New Oxford Street
London
WC1A 1AH.

The Terrence Higgins Trust Limited
BM AIDS
London
WC1N 3XX.

Both the above organizations provide leaflets on AIDS that are regularly updated. Some of them are free.

British Association for Counselling (BAC)
37a Sheep Street
Rugby
Warwickshire
CV21 3BX.
Telephone: 0788 78328/9

BAC can provide names of specialist counsellors.

Useful telephone numbers

Terrence Higgins Trust Limited Helpline – 01 833 2970 (7pm–10pm every day)

College of Health – 01 980 4848 (6pm–10pm every day).
12 different tapes on different aspects of AIDS.

Healthlines/AIDSlines – Some areas have set up Healthlines or AIDSlines. Ask British Telecom in your area.

Local Health Education/Promotion Units can provide information, teaching resources, and in-service training. Contact the District Health Authority for address and phone number.

London Friend – 01 359 7371 (7pm–10pm every day).
A befriending and counselling agency dealing with gay and bisexual men and women.
Note: Friend exists in most other major cities in the UK, and local telephone numbers can be found in the local telephone directory or from the Citizens Advice Bureaux.

London Gay Switchboard – 01 837 7324 (24 hours every day).
Note: Gay Switchboards exist in several other large towns and will be
found in the local telephone directory, or their number can be
obtained from London Gay Switchboard.

GUM (Genito-urinary medicine) clinics exist in all NHS hospitals, and
their telephone numbers and addresses are available from your Local
Health Authority. They may be in the telephone directory under
Venereal or Sexually Transmitted Diseases. The nearest hospital can also
give you the information.

Sources of further information

Scutari Marketing
PO Box 8,
Leigh,
Lancashire WN7 1HU
Telephone: 0942 261001
(AIDS guidelines
AIDS package – book and tape)

UKCC
Distribution Office
23, Portland Place,
London, W1N 3AF
Telephone: 01 637 7181
AIDS and HIV infection
Circular PC/88/03
Circulars and videos are also available from the Department of Health.

10

Research in general practice

INTRODUCTION

Research is the method used to determine facts about a subject. The method is a planned step-by-step process. The process can be divided into four stages.

- Stage One: asking questions;
- Stage Two: planning the research;
- Stage Three: analysing and interpreting the findings;
- Stage Four: presenting of the facts.

This chapter will focus on stages one and two of the research process. Further reading for the remainder of the process is listed at the end of the chapter.

Stage one in the research process

Asking questions

It is possible to ask questions about anything, but not all questions are suitable for research. The following are the essential characteristics of a research question:

- the question should be important, relevant and significant enough that an answer is necessary;
- the question asked should be interesting, not only to the researcher, but also to those helping and participating in the study;
- the question should be answerable within a reasonable length of time, not only to maintain motivation of those involved in

the research but also because criteria relating to the study may change.

Selecting questions

As a question is asked or thought of it should be written down and filed away in subject order using an index system. These questions should be reviewed periodically, say monthly. Some of the questions will need to be discarded, others revised and some questions may need to be explored further.

Stage two: planning the research project

Planning the project takes considerable time and is a very important part of the research. This stage should not be hurried.

Formulating an idea

Having decided on the question to be answered, the answer to that question should be predicted and the results that would be needed to support that answer noted.

The idea should be developed around the question to be answered, making notes of the aims and plans at the same time. This stage should be left untouched for a few weeks and then returned to, checking it over and making changes as necessary.

It is important to take advice and views from friends and colleagues in the early stages of planning. Speaking to those who have experience in the area to be investigated, or who have research experience, can be invaluable at the embryonic stage of the project.

Next it is necessary to review and search the literature; list the resources to be checked, and start simply and generally by gathering information from the medical/nursing journal with which you are familiar. Collect a year's bound volumes and go through the index looking for the subject area of the proposed research.

While you are scanning the literature in this general way, note any article of interest to the proposed area of research with details of author's name, where the work was done, the journal's date, volume number and page numbers. Aim to collect 15–20 references and be prepared to go back another year through the journals for references if necessary.

Having started with a familiar journal, repeat the exercise by searching the indexes of other journals, reading the relevant articles and making notes on cards summarizing them, along with details of author(s), pages, volume, year, title and name of journal.

Your literature search should also include Government reports; you should note, too, that a number of libraries will undertake a search on your behalf. However, reference lists and abstracting services are no substitute for personal reading.

The aims of the research project

Having asked the question, considered what the answer might be, and what information would be needed to substantiate the answer, and having explored the literature, the aims of the project are the next step.

Ideas which have previously been thought through now need to be put down in the form of aims and objectives so that plans may be formulated to achieve a relevant result.

An hypothesis is a term which can be used instead of 'aim and objectives'. The Shorter Oxford Dictionary defines a hypothesis as '...a supposition in general; something assumed to be true without proof'. With a hypothesis clearly stated, the research which follows seeks to prove or disprove the assumption.

Research design

Planning and designing a research project is like putting a recipe together. The person undertaking the research needs to describe in detail the ingredients for the recipe, their preparation and the way they are to be used. Detailed planning at this stage will assist in the analysis of the results.

The subject

Numerator is the term used for what is to be studied, and how it is to be defined.

Denominator is the term used for stating from where the information will be collected.

Sample

A sample is part of a whole, and a carefully drawn sample should reflect the whole. This can be either a **stratified sample** where various groups in the whole population are separated out before the sample is taken; or a **random sample** in which each person in the population has an equal chance of being chosen.

In general practice there are a number of aids from which samples may be readily obtained:

- The patient's medical record;
- The age-sex register;
- A self-constructed disease index;
- The practice computer;
- Data from repeat prescriptions;
- Via consultations.

Types of research

Retrospective research analyses data already available. It means that information has not been collected with a particular project in mind. On the other hand, **prospective research** aims to collect data with the project directly in mind.

Methods of collecting information

Once the numerator and denominator have been decided upon, and a broad outline of the study planned, the methods of collecting data need to be decided upon. It is of importance that the technique decided upon is valid and reliable. A valid method is one which measures what it sets out to measure. A reliable method is one which produces repeatable results.

Figure 10.1 summarizes methods for collecting data in general practice.

The size of the study

Decisions have to be made about how large the study will be, and how long the study should last.

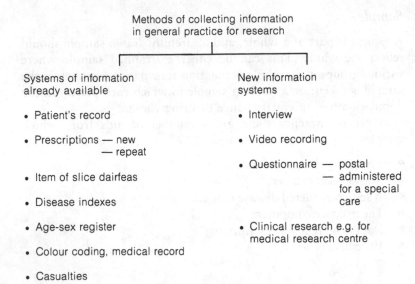

Figure 10.1 Methods of collecting information in general practice for research.

Ethics in research

The following issues need to be considered under this heading: confidentiality; informed consent; and the use of placebos or controls in clinical trials. The support of an ethical committee and the Local Medical Committee may need to be sought.

Research protocol

The research protocol puts on paper the proposals of the study. This statement needs to include the following:

1. Introduction;
2. Review of the literature;
3. Aims and objectives of the study or the hypothesis;
4. Methods of collecting the data;
5. Methods proposed for the analysis of the information;
6. Financial implications and support needed;
7. Copies of any questionnaires or other forms for collecting data;
8. References;
9. Curriculum vitae of person undertaking the research.

ESSENTIAL STEPS TO BE FOLLOWED IN THE RESEARCH PROCESS

1. Ask the questions;
2. Predict the answer to the question posed;
3. Determine what information is needed to support the answer;
4. Explore the literature around the subject;
5. State the aims and the objectives of the project or state the hypothesis of the study;
6. Plan the research to
   (a) achieve the aims and objectives
   (b) to disprove or prove the assumption stated in the hypothesis.

INGREDIENTS OF THE PLAN

1. Numerator;
2. Denominator;
3. Sample;
4. Types of research ie. retrospective or prospective;
5. Methods of collecting information;
6. Analyse the data from the information collected;
7. Interpret the results;
8. Present the facts.

FURTHER READING

Bennett, A.E. and Ritchie, K. (1975) *Questionnaires in Medicine*, Oxford University Press, London.

Carmines, E. and Zeller, R. (1979) *Reliability and Validity Assessment*, Sage Publications, London.

de Bono, E. (1976) *The Use of Lateral Thinking*, Cape, London.

Fox, D.J. (1976) *Fundamentals of Research in Nursing*. Appleton-Century-Crofts, New York.

Health Education Council (1984) *Research Handbook*. Health Education Council, London.

Huff, D. (1973) *How to Lie with Statistics*. Penguin.

Long, A.F. (1984) *Research into Health and Illness: Issues in Design, Analysis and Practice*. Gower Publications, Aldershot.

Moser, C. and Kalton, G. (1972) *Survey Methods in Social Investigation*, Heinemann, London.

Polit, D.F. and Hungler, B.P. (1983) *Nursing Research: Principles and Methods*, J.P. Lippincott Co., Philadelphia.

Reid, N.G. and Boore, J.R.P. (1987) *Research Methods and Statistics in Health Care*, Edward Arnold, London.

Rowntree, D. (1981) *Statistics without Tears*, Penguin.

Seaman, C.C. and Verhonick, P.J. (1982) *Research Methods for Undergraduate Students in Nursing*, Appleton-Century-Crofts, New York.

APPENDIX

Useful addresses

National groups and associations

Action against Allergy Association
43 The Downs,
London, SW20 8HG.

Action on Smoking and Health (ASH)
5–11 Mortimer Street,
London, W1N 7RH.

Age Concern
England: Bernard Sunley House,
60 Pitcarn Road,
Mitcham, Surrey.
N. Ireland: N. Ireland Old People's Welfare Council,
128 Gt Victoria Street,
Belfast, BT2 7BG.
Scotland: Scottish Old People's Welfare Council,
33 Castle Street,
Edinburgh, EH2 3DN.
Wales: 1 Park Grove Cardiff, CF1 3BJ.

Artsline (Arts for Disabled)
5 Crowndale Road,
London, NW1 1TU.

Association for One Parent Families (Gingerbread)
35 Wellington Street,
London, WC2E 7BN.

Asthma Research Council
300 Upper Street,
London, N1 2XX.

Association of Swimming Therapy (AST)
Treetops,
Swan Hill,
Ellesmere,
Salop SY 12 OLZ.

Back Pain Association
31–33 Park Road,
Teddington,
Middlesex TW11 OAB.

British Agencies for Adoption and Fostering (BAAF),
11 Southwark Street,
London, SE1 1RQ.

British Diabetic Association
10 Queen Anne Street,
London, W1M OBD.

British Dyslexia Association
Church Lane,
Peppard,
Oxon, RG9 5JN.

British Heart Foundation
102 Gloucester Place,
London, W1H 4DH.

British Migraine Association
178A High Road,
Byfleet,
Weybridge,
Surrey KT14 7ED.

British Pregnancy Advisory Service (BPAS)
Austy Manor,
Wootton Wawen,
Solihull,
West Midlands.

British Sports Association for the Disabled
Haywood House,
Barnard Crescent,
Aylesbury Park,
Bucks. HP21 9PP.

Cancer Relief
Michael Sobell House,

30 Dorset Square,
London, NW1 6QL.

Colostomy Welfare Group
38–39 Eccleston Square,
London, SW1V 1PB.

CRUSE, National Organisation for the Widowed and their Children,
Cruse House,
126 Sheen Road,
Richmond,
Surrey, TW9 1UR.

Down's Syndrome Association
CBI Centrepoint,
103 New Oxford Street,
London, WC1A 1DU.

Gamblers Anonymous
17/23 Blantyre Street,
Cheyne Walk,
London, SW10.

Haemophilia Society
PO Box 9,
16 Trinity Street,
London, SE1 1DE.

Marriage Guidance
Herbert Gray College,
Little Church Street,
Rugby CV21 3AP.

Mastectomy Association
26 Harrison Street,
Kings Cross,
London WC1 8JG.

National Council for One Parent Families
255 Kentish Town Road,
London, NW5 2LX.

Royal Society for Mentally Handicapped Children and Adults
(MENCAP)
RSMHCA Centre,
123 Golden Lane,
London, EC1Y ORT.

Professional bodies

United Kingdom Central Council for Nursing, Midwifery and Health Visiting,
23 Portland Place,
London, W1.

English National Board for Nursing, Midwifery and Health Visiting,
170 Tottenham Court Road,
London, W1.

Royal College of Nursing of the United Kingdom,
20 Cavendish Square,
London, W1.

Royal College of Nursing of the United Kingdom,
Subscriptions,
Glynteg House,
Station Terrace,
Ely
Cardiff, CF5 4XG.

Royal College of General Practitioners
14 Princes Gate,
London, SW7.

British Medical Association,
BMA House,
Tavistock Square,
London, WC1.

Medical Defence Union,
3 Devonshire Place,
London, W1 9JB

Medical Research Council,
20 Park Crescent,
London, W1.

The British Library,
2 Sheraton Street,
London, W1.

Index

Printed in the United States
by Baker & Taylor Publisher Services

Printed in the United States
by Baker & Taylor Publisher Services